CLINICAL
INTERVIEWING SKILLS

*A programmed manual for data gathering,
evaluation, and patient management*

LON A. HOOVER, D. O.

Michigan State University
Department of Family Medicine
College of Osteopathic Medicine
Fee Hall
East Lansing, MI 48824

CLINICAL INTERVIEWING SKILLS

A programmed manual for data gathering, evaluation, and patient management

ROBERT E. FROELICH, M.D., F.A.P.A.

Professor and Chairman of Psychiatry, School of Primary Medical Care, The University of Alabama in Huntsville, Huntsville, Alabama

F. MARIAN BISHOP, Ph.D., M.S.P.H.

Professor and Chairman of Community Medicine, School of Primary Medical Care, The University of Alabama in Huntsville, Huntsville, Alabama

THIRD EDITION

THE C. V. MOSBY COMPANY

Saint Louis   1977

THIRD EDITION

Copyright © 1977 by The C. V. Mosby Company

All rights reserved. No part of this book may be reproduced
in any manner without written permission of the publisher.

Previous editions copyrighted 1969, 1972

Printed in the United States of America

Distributed in Great Britain by Henry Kimpton, London

The C. V. Mosby Company
11830 Westline Industrial Drive, St. Louis, Missouri 63141

Library of Congress Cataloging in Publication Data

Froelich, Robert E   1929-
    Clinical interviewing skills.

    Published in 1969 under title: Medical interviewing.
    Includes index.
    1. Medical history taking. I. Bishop, F
Marian, joint author. II. Title.
RC65.F7   1977   616.07'5   76-62992
ISBN 0-8016-1702-2

VH/VH/VH   9   8   7   6   5   4   3   2   1

INTRODUCTION

To the health professional, regardless of the type of practice, the ability to establish a satisfactory professional-patient relationship rests on the use of communication skills in the interview. This manual is intended to teach the student basic skills of interviewing through active involvement with simulated patient contact. Because of the increasing number of students and the limited number of faculty available to teach interviewing, some method of self-study and simulation of actual experience is needed.

Although all persons communicate, the ability to communicate skillfully and purposefully with the other person rarely occurs naturally. It is a common misunderstanding that the awarding of a degree also confers the ability to communicate and to elicit information and responses from others. No degree guarantees this skill. Our national examinations for certification and honor (examples are the national boards in medicine, specialty certification boards, and International Transactional Analysis Association) are now focusing more and more on the presentation of taped interviews, live interviews before examiners, and simulated interviews to measure the interviewing skills of the applicants. Knowledge, practice, and experience with meaningful feedback are required to develop precise, predictable, effective, and satisfying techniques of communication and to master the many techniques of interviewing.

Question: What makes a good interviewer (therapist)?

Answer: A number of studies over the last decade are coming forth with three basic qualities of the good or successful therapist. It follows that a good interviewer will have the same qualities since therapy depends on successful data gathering and upon a successful relationship between the health professional and patient.

1. The good interviewer is appropriately nurturant. By this is meant that the professional is supportive and helpful so that the patient grows in strength. Overly nurturant care would tend to keep the patient functioning at an immature, inadequate level requiring continued support. Inadequate nurturant care would tend to let the patient struggle with the solution of a problem alone to the point that the patient may give up or not succeed in solving the problem.

2. The good interviewer conveys to the patient a conceptual model by which the patient can understand his or her illness, problem, or disease. In the good interview the conceptual model is conveyed by example and meaningful illustration rather than by lecturing the patient, having the patient read material, or sending the patient to a class. The key check to whether or not you have been successful in conveying a model to the patient is to learn how the patient understands his or her disease, illness, or problem.

3. The good interviewer involves the patient in the problem-solving process. The patient is increasingly responsible for giving the data, for seeking the solution, for establishing the relationship, and for following the directions necessary to carry out the treatment.

In the minds of most patients competence and interest in the patient are inseparable. The feeling of disinterest implies to the patient that the interviewer is not motivated to exercise scientific competency. Is it possible that much apparent lack of interest is, in reality, a lack of interviewing skills? If so, it would be negligent not to rectify this gross defect.

Skill and time are two related components of a successful patient interview. The more skillful the interviewer, the less time required for an interview. If the practical limitations of time pose problems for the busy health professional, it becomes even more imperative that skills be perfected for directing and guiding the interview. The professional must be sufficiently skilled so that even under pressures he or she can establish and maintain an unhurried, interested manner. The patient must feel that he or she is receiving the professional's undivided attention and energy throughout the interview.

A good interview provides a direct path to understanding the patient's difficulties. Symptoms often appear long before the current laboratory tests are capable of detecting disordered physiology. A careful, detailed, properly analyzed and interpreted history can usually lead the interviewer to an accurate diagnosis and successful treatment plan. Furthermore, the interview may establish a therapeutic relationship that motivates the patient toward cooperation with the interviewer.

A complete interview and the recording of the history are very costly procedures. Therefore, they must be accomplished efficiently and in a manner personally satisfying to both the interviewer and the patient. The traditional methods of obtaining and recording a patient's history that persist in teaching hospitals are used rarely in either the office practice or the hospital practice because the cost to the patient is prohibitive.

As we observe students in their initial interviewing, two major flaws are evident. First, most students utilize only a few of the many alternatives available to them in guiding an interview and in responding to a patient. The predominant technique is to ask direct, specific questions. Second, most students do not know what information to seek next. The interview tends to jump illogically from topic to topic, depending on the next question that can be recalled. *This manual is intended to actively teach the student alternative ways of responding to a patient and to develop a feeling for the appropriate lead.*

In our teaching experiences with students we have been, and continue to be, impressed with their eagerness to conduct a good interview. We are also sympathetic to the reluctance on the part of any student to experiment and practice the various interviewing skills with an assigned patient, especially since such interviewing must often be carried out in the presence of other patients. We believe that simulated patient contact will allow the student some advance experimentation and practice that can be conducted in privacy and at an individual pace.

Question: How would you define an interview? How would it differ from a social interaction?

Answer: An interview is a communication between two or more people with a purpose to which both (or all) agree. There are two socially defined roles: the interviewer and the interviewee. The interview is to focus on the interviewee, usually to help the interviewee in some way, and to obtain information from (and occasionally to give information to) the interviewee. A social interaction differs in that the roles are not necessarily defined as above, the focus is usually mutually shared by each participant, and the purpose is not necessarily defined.

Question: What is a history? How does it differ from an interview?

Answer: A history is the *organization* of information obtained from a patient. The interview and the history differ primarily in the organization of the information.

In order to obtain reliable information from a patient in an efficient manner, the interviewer must direct the patient to information in an area closely associated with the current thoughts of the patient. If the interviewer jumps from topic to topic, the patient has a difficult time following the conversation, the interview contains many pauses while the patient thinks about what the interviewer is asking, and the flow of information is very slow. On the other hand, if the interviewer stays with a topic until all of the relevant information is obtained, the flow of information is more rapid, the patient is ready for the next question, and the patient spontaneously remembers more details that may give the needed differential diagnostic clues.

Usually the interviewer seeks information related to an organ system, a symptom, a period in the patient's life (specific hour, day, or year), a feeling, or a thought before going to a new topic. In writing or reporting the history the interviewer may organize the information around a diagnosis, presenting information from different times, organ systems, or symptoms in order to lead the reader or listener to the diagnosis while listing the differential diagnostic information.

In the last 15 years many procedures have been developed for teaching interviewing techniques. Little focus on interviewing skills occurs in the literature prior to the 1960's. Since then, there has been a great deal of interest in the field, with resultant input from many fine teachers. In addition to the body of this text, there are additional suggestions in the Appendix to aid in the learning of interviewing skills by the student.

CONTENTS

PART ONE

CONDUCTING THE INTERVIEW

CHAPTER 1

PREPARATION FOR AN INTERVIEW

GENERAL CONSIDERATIONS

Each interview has a manifest purpose and goal. In addition, there will be latent purposes and goals that may or may not be immediately evident. The more common and obvious manifest goals are to gain information, establish a relationship, obtain an understanding in one or both parties involved in the interview, and to lend support or direction to one of the parties.

Question: How does an interview differ from helping a person fill out a questionnaire?

Answer: The most important difference is that the interview "makes meaning" out of what the other person says. In the questionnaire the respondent's answer to the question is accepted at face value. No attempt is made on most questionnaires to obtain further elaboration and meaning to the answer. In the interview the respondent's answer is considered, amplified, elaborated, and questioned until both parties arrive at nearly the same understanding of what was meant by the response.

From this question and answer it is suggested that an interview is not really fulfilling its purpose if the respondent's answers are not elaborated, clarified, and made meaningful. We concur with this suggestion. When the primary purpose of the interview is to obtain information, then it does not make sense to waste time in an interview if a questionnaire will accomplish the same goal. In many situations, interviews have been replaced with questionnaires or with computer interviews. In a few situations the substitution has been acceptable, but in the vast majority of situations the substitution has been unacceptable. However, in situations in which it is important to have an accurate interpretation of the information given, the interview has stood the test of time.

From this background it is clear that the focus of this text needs to be on the collection of meaningful information rather than just obtaining information whose meaning is open to each reader's interpretation.

3

PURPOSE OF AN INTERVIEW

The areas vital to successful interviewing and patient management are obtaining information about the history of the patient, establishing rapport, understanding the patient's reactions in the present, and understanding the total patient. Difficult management may result from a deficiency in any of these areas. The purpose of the interview is fourfold:

1. To gather information about the patient and his/her illness that is not available from other sources
2. To establish a relationship with the patient that will facilitate diagnosis and treatment
3. To give the patient an understanding of his/her illness
4. To support and direct the patient in his/her treatment

Question: Can an interview be replaced with a questionnaire or a computer programmed to obtain information about the patient and his/her illness?

Answer: Questionnaires and computer programs can obtain some information. They have an effect on the relationship that is established which varies with the individual patient and with the setting. So far, such questionnaires and computer programs have not been programmed either to help the patient understand his/her illness or to support and direct the patient in his/her treatment. In addition, the questionnaire and computer programs do not have the ability to "make meaning" out the response of the patient.

Only in the interview can terminology be clarified. The meaning of pain to a patient and the degree to which he/she feels it cannot be obtained from our present forms on which patients record their history. Such shades of meaning are difficult to understand even when obtained firsthand from the patient who is experiencing the pain. When the information is obtained secondhand via a printed form, it is still more difficult to understand.

The word *pain* is to the unique sensation that the patient is experiencing as a map is to a territory. The word is a symbolic representation of the territory; it is not the territory, and the interviewer's concept of the sensation as a result of hearing the word *pain* may not be the same as that being experienced by the patient. Only in the interview can the interviewer's concept be clarified.

The difference between what we *mean* to say, what we *do* say, and how another person *interprets* what we say often is a surprise to students. If you have had little experience with word meaning, do the following exercise and see what you can learn. Then follow the exercise with a discussion of what each of you learned. The rules of the exercise are:

1. Person A makes a statement to person B. The statement can be about anything and should have some significance to person A; for example, "I would like to know you better."
2. Person B asks questions of person A as follows: "By that do you mean . . ." Person B completes the question in any way he/she chooses.
3. Person A can answer *only* with "yes" or "no".
4. Person B must obtain three "yes" answers.

This exercise is referred to as a "make meaning" exercise and has been most productive when we have used it with various health professionals and followed it with a discussion of what each had learned.

In the exercise you may have noted that you used some nonverbal clues to guide you to an understanding of the meaning of the message from A. You will understand the principles involved in this exercise when you give directions to patients. If you remember that the "message is in the receiver," you will inquire of the patient what he/she heard you say and what that means to him/her. In checking out what the patient heard, one learns frequently that the patient was more tuned to nonverbal messages from you than to the words that you were using.

Question: A health professional was recently overheard taking a history. He spent almost all of his time asking specific questions that required one or two words to answer. Which of the four purposes of the interview did the interviewer fulfill?
A. To gather information about the patient and his/her illness that is not available from other sources.
B. To establish a relationship with the patient that will facilitate diagnosis and treatment.
C. To give the patient an understanding of his/her illness.
D. To support and direct the patient in his/her treatment.

Answer: The correct answer is A, since he may have obtained the information needed, but he established a relationship that does *not* usually facilitate diagnosis, treatment, or understanding. Specific questions neither assist the patient to understand his illness nor lend support to him, thus negating B, C, and D.

By answering a series of specific questions, the patient is forced to remain passive and dependent upon the interviewer. The patient is not permitted to accept any responsibility for his/her history and will probably continue in the same dependent role throughout treatment. Furthermore, when 80% of the time is spent by the interviewer asking questions and the patient is talking only 20% of the time, the information learned from the patient per unit of time is very little. The interview process in this example is not efficient.

Question: In an interview information can be obtained that is difficult or impossible to obtain from any other source. You are able to obtain detailed information about the illness that is not available from any source other than the _____.

Answer: patient.

You are also able to learn how the patient feels about his/her illness, how the patient feels while telling you about the illness, how he/she relates to you, and something about the kind of a person the patient is. This behavioral information will be useful to you in planning and carrying out the patient's treatment.

Information about an illness (such as reaction to previous medical care) that is charged with emotion is not readily available from sources other than the interview. The emotionally charged information is not usually given to the office receptionist or secretary. There are times, however, when emotionally charged information is available from members of the family and from another professional persons, such as a social worker, psychologist, pastor, or nurse.

The interview, when properly conducted, is the hub of medical care. All aspects of care revolve around it. To carry this line of reasoning one step further, the medical care of a patient disintegrates when it is not held together with a properly conducted interview and the professional relationship developed by the interview.

The interviewer must fulfill four basic requirements to conduct a successful interview:

1. Know what information is needed.
2. Know how to get the information.
3. Have a plan, a flexible order, for obtaining the information.
4. Guide, but not dominate, the interview.

Question: The interviewer's time is scheduled. He/she usually knows how much time is allotted for each patient. One resident said, "I just get them started talking and then pick out from what they say what I believe to be important."

    A. Who has more control of the interview, the resident or the patient?

    B. Why is it unlikely that this resident will obtain the information he/she needs in the time allotted?

Answer: A. The patient, because he/she can choose what he/she wishes to talk about.

    B. The resident may have to wait a long time to get the information necessary to make a differential diagnosis, whereas in a guided interview, there would be direction for the patient's attention to the topic critical for diagnosis. In addition, the interviewer's active guidance shows an interest in the patient.

Guiding an interview is not a difficult task. The major problem is knowing what to do. The section on practice interviews (p. 89) presents information to help you guide an interview.

PREINTERVIEW DATA

Question: A patient was ushered into the office by the assistant. In a moment the interviewer entered and said, "Hello, Mr. Jones." The patient replied, "I am not Mr. Jones, I am John Kline." How would you, as the patient, feel?

What should the interviewer have done before entering the office?

Answer: You would probably feel let down. You might assume that the interviewer did not have the courtesy or did not care enough about you to know your name.

The interviewer should have some information about the patient, including his/her name, before entering the interviewing room.

As a minimum, an interviewer should have the following information before seeing the patient:

Name
Address (local or out-of-town; what neighborhood, if in town)
Sex
Age
Occupation and religion
Reason for visit, or referral note
Whether or not previous records are available
Name of previous health professional (if any)

The above list of information is usually obtained by the office receptionist or secretary, clinic admission office, or hospital ward secretary and is available even in the emergency room.

Question: A physician entered the office to see a patient and said, "Hello, Mr. Kline. I am Dr. Armstrong." The patient responded, "Yes, Doctor, I remember you. I saw you last March for my employment physical."
What is the patient saying to the physician?
How would you feel if you were the patient?
What did the doctor omit in his preparation for the interview?

Answer: The patient is asking the physician if he doesn't remember the visit last March. As a patient you may quickly feel that the doctor has a limited interest in you, both as a patient and as a person. The doctor and his staff failed to check whether or not there was a record on this patient and the date of his last visit.

Question: A physician greeted a new patient with, "Howdy, George, I'm Dr. Armstrong." The patient is the president of the largest bank in Detroit and is on vacation at the Lake of the Ozarks. How might this patient be expected to react to this greeting that is overly familiar in a professional setting?

Answer: He might feel that he had picked a "hayseed" for a doctor and would seek to conclude the visit as soon as possible.

An observant, perceptive office assistant can inform the interviewer, before he/she sees the patient, about such facts as the patient's personality, emotional state, and reaction to illness as noted in his/her contact with the patient. The assistant may also note changes he/she perceives from visit to visit. These observations are most important to the interviewer as a validation of his/her own observations.

Question: In addition to the above observations, the interviewer should

have noted George's _____ and _____
before entering the office.

Answer: occupation and address

In addition to giving the interviewer the needed background information and notes from the assistant's observations of the patient, an interviewer will sometimes instruct the assistant to introduce him/her to a new patient.

SOURCES OF DATA

Information about the patient and his/her illness comes from a number of possible sources:

Referral letter, note, or telephone communication
Questionnaire filled out by the patient
Patient's record (office and hospital)
Secretary or assistant
Social worker, counselors, referral agencies, employers, pastors
Patient's family
School and work records

Not every source of information is relevant to every patient, but over a number of interviews all sources of information will be important to the interviewer at some time.

Question: A 45-year-old career Master Sergeant in the army had an acute myocardial infarction while his son was home from the navy. The sergeant's recovery was prolonged and stormy. He constantly required more than the normal amount of sedatives and tranquilizers. After his recovery, information was obtained that could have been used to reduce the workload on his heart during his recovery. What error did the staff make?

Answer: The staff failed to get sufficient information about the patient to understand properly why he had the heart attack when he did. If the staff had talked with the patient's family, they would have learned that the patient (several hours before his heart attack) was acutely upset when he learned that his son was A.W.O.L. from the navy. Had the staff obtained this information, the patient's feelings (such as rage, fear, and anxiety) could have been dealt with and his recovery could have been subsequently hastened. By proper interviewing the information about the son would have been known by the staff.

Question: A patient had recently been evaluated for loss of sensation in his legs as the result of lead poisoning. The loss of sensation persisted and a few weeks later a relative brought him to the same hospital emergency room of a university hospital with a foot laceration. The attending physician treated the wound, bandaged it, and instructed the patient to call or return immediately if pain developed in the foot. The patient was told he should come back in 3 days. Upon his return in 3 days, the patient's toes showed signs of swelling and infection. What error did the physician make?

Answer: The physician failed to obtain a history of the previous illness from either the hospital chart, the patient, or the relative who brought him to the emergency room. Any of these sources would have indicated that pain sensations in the patient's foot could not be relied upon to judge whether or not the bandage was too tight and interfering with circulation.

CHAPTER 2

INITIATING THE INTERVIEW

A patient may visit the health professional for a variety of reasons that range from acute symptoms to routine check-ups to getting advice concerning a problem in the family. Each of these reasons will require a different approach to the interview. This section deals primarily with initial interviews; however, the techniques learned here are useful in other types of patient encounters.

OPENING STATEMENT

Question: Formulate your opening remarks for the following situation: Mrs. Arnold is waiting in the reception room. The record indicates that Mrs. Arnold is 35 years old, the mother of three children, lives in town, was referred to you by Mrs. Jackson, and has requested this first visit because of a dull pain in the left side of her head. It is obvious that Mrs. Arnold is anxious and concerned about her discomfort.

Answer: The opening remarks would be something like the following: Mrs. Arnold? I am . . . (your name).

The opening statement in initiating the history is important. It sets the tone of the professional relationship as well as the direction of the interview.

Question: Which of the following questions would *not* be appropriate in this situation?
A. How do you like this weather?
B. What troubles are you having?
C. I see you live in town; how long have you lived here?
D. Have you known Mrs. Jackson a long time?
E. What is the situation that brings you here today?

Answer: A, C, and D. These questions have the quality of breaking the ice, and they are used to put the patient at ease. But the question is raised as to whether a patient who is paying for your time wants to spend part of it talking about one of these topics. Another objection to these choices is that they do not set the stage for a professional relationship. These questions would be appropriate in many nonprofessional settings.

Even though you may have information about the patient, you must learn from the patient directly why he/she has come.

Question: Which of the following openings would you choose to elicit this information from Mrs. Arnold?
  A. The information I have indicates you have a dull pain on the side of your head. Tell me about it.
  B. What troubles are you having?
  C. What is the situation that brings you here today?
  D. You have a dull pain on the side of your head?
  E. How are things?

Answer: B and C give the patient freedom and define the area of discussion.
  A and D restrict the patient's response to the topic she reported to the assistant. Frequently, a patient will initially give a reason for the visit (sometimes referred to as an "admission ticket") that is a partial truth. Immediate exploration limited to the "admission ticket" may obscure the real reason for the visit. E gives the patient a great deal of freedom, but it does not differentiate the interview from a social visit.

Once the patient has given information to an office member other than yourself, you need to let the patient know what you know about him/her. By stating what you know at the beginning of an interview in a frank and honest manner, you show interest in the information the patient has given and encourage a forthright relationship. The following combination of A and C is a suggested opening to Mrs. Arnold:

I am _____. I understand that you have a dull pain on the side of your head. What is the situation?

With this opening statement, Mrs. Arnold is not limited to discussing her pain, but is free to begin the interview in any manner she chooses. In addition, you have honestly shared and checked your information with her, allowing for immediate correction of any misunderstandings.

The receptionist indicates that Mr. Glenn has come to the office because of a sore back. As he sits down you notice that he is very cautious in using his left leg in lowering himself into the chair.

Question: Write your opening statement.

Answer: Compare your response with the following:

Mr. Glenn, I am _____. The assistant tells me that you have a sore back. What is the situation?

It is tempting to call attention to your astute observation and ask about his left leg. This action would direct his immediate response to his left leg, however, without giving him an opportunity to discuss another topic of perhaps greater concern. You can always ask about the left leg later if he does not mention it.

THERAPEUTIC CONTRACTS

For every relationship between two persons there are either spoken or unspoken rules that make up the agreement or contract. The health professional–patient interview is no exception. In fact, there are usually three contracts established in the course of treating a patient. The health professional and patient agree (1) to relate, (2) to exchange information, and (3) to give and receive treatment. When the staff and the patient do not agree on the terms of these contracts, the results are misleading communications, anger, and misunderstandings.

Question: You ask a patient what the trouble is, and the patient responds with, "That is what I came to you to find out." What is the implied contract?

Answer: The usual professional-patient contract is not accepted by this patient. The patient is deviating from the usual patient role by neither giving information freely nor helping you understand what troubles him. In such a situation, you must decide whether or not to accept the patient's implied contract of not giving information and continue to deal with this resistant (dependent) patient or whether the patient can be helped to modify his position.

> If you do not accept the contract implied by the patient in this example, you must discuss the situation with the patient and establish a contract to which both of you can agree. If a compromise cannot be reached, a last resort may be for the patient to find another health professional.

> The implied contract is, "Take care of me. Don't ask me to take any responsibility for my care."

The contract of the therapeutic relationship is defined by a discussion concerning what the patient expects and wants from the relationship and what the health professional is able and willing to offer. (See example on pp. 144 and 149.)

FACILITATION AND OPEN-ENDED QUESTIONS

facilitation a verbal or nonverbal communication that encourages the patient to say more, yet does not specify the area or topic to be discussed.

open-ended question a question asking for information from the patient and specifying the content in general terms.*

Question: Which of the following are facilitations:
A. How are things?
B. Uh huh!
C. What troubles are you having?
D. You have been having pain in your jaw? Tell me about it.

Answer: A and B
C and D are an open-ended question and an open-ended response that specify the area to be discussed—troubles and pain in jaw. C and D give the patient freedom in his/her reply but differ from a facilitation by giving some structure to the answer.

_____

*Blyth, J. W., and Alter, M.: How to conduct a selection interview, Los Angeles, 1965, Sherbourne Press, p. 344.

Other examples of open-ended questions are, "What brings you to see me?" "How did it happen?"

Open-ended questions and facilitations are useful to open an interview and to follow the patient's opening of a new topic. Early in the discussion of a topic you want to know the following:

How the patient views the topic.

What the patient thinks is related and important to the topic.

How much the patient can tell you about the topic on his/her own before you question him/her more actively.

Question: A patient points to his left wrist and says to you, "You know, last week I had a pain right here in my wrist." This is the first time you have heard about any symptoms related to this patient's wrist. What is your response?

Answer: Examples of a facilitation or an open-ended question you might have chosen are:

Uh huh! (Facilitation)

What can you recall about it? (Open-ended question)

What was it like? (Open-ended question)

Tell me about it. (Open-ended statement)

In the middle of an interview a patient tells you that he has some pain while walking. You want to know more about it.

Question: Write out your response to this patient. What type of response will you make?

Answer: What did you notice about it? (Open-ended question)

Silence with an expression which says, "I am interested, tell me more." (Facilitation)

CHAPTER 3

ASSISTING·THE PATIENT'S NARRATIVE

SUPPORT, EMPATHY, AND REASSURANCE

support   a response that shows interest in, concern for, or understanding of the patient.*

reassurance   a response that tends to establish the sense of merit, well-being, or self-reliance in the patient.†

empathy   a response that recognizes or names the patient's feeling and does not in any way critize it; accepts the feeling in the patient even though the interviewer may believe the feeling to be wrong.

Question: Reassurance, support, and empathy are three somewhat similar types of responses made by interviewers. All three deal with

the _____ of the patient rather than with the literal meaning of what he/she is saying.

Answer: feelings

Each patient maintains within him/herself a feeling of well-being, of being acceptable to him/herself and others, and of meeting certain standards of behavior. The manifestations of the patient's attempts to maintain a feeling of "goodness" are in opposition to divulging information that exposes his/her failures, weaknesses (as the patient views them), and inability to perform expected tasks. A feeling of being defective may interfere with the patient's ability to share openly his/her symptoms with the professional. The professional uses empathy, support, reassurance, and a noncritical approach to penetrate this natural resistance or defense.

Reassurance

Reassurance can be used to decrease the patient's resistance to discussing a topic. A patient says, "I shouldn't complain about this pain, but I just can't stand the constant ache."

---

*Enelow, A. J., and Wexler, M.: Psychiatry in the practice of medicine, New York, 1966, Oxford University Press, Inc., pp. 59-60.
†Verwoerdt, A.: Communication with the fatally ill, Springfield, Ill., 1966, Charles C Thomas, Publisher, pp. 34-37.

Question: How would you let the patient know that you understand the severe pain he/she is in?

Answer: Compare your response to the following:
That pain is enough to get to anyone.
It's hard to take when there is no relief.
That kind of pain is hard to take when there is no relief.
A constant pain is very disturbing. (I understand.)

A patient says, "My wife gets tired of my soft diet and every now and then fixes me something that tears up my stomach. Then I go back on a full dose of medicine. In a few days I get comfortable. If only I could get back to normal and not be concerned about what I eat."

Question: Make up a response showing that you understand this patient's impatience.

Answers: Compare your response to the following:
After this length of time it wears your patience thin.
It would surely be nice to be able to enjoy some pizza and beer again, wouldn't it?
It really tests your patience, doesn't it?

As a professional, you are often called on to offer reassurance (restore confidence) to the patient in panic. You give this reassurance nonverbally, by being calm yourself. Since distress and anxiety are contagious, manipulation of the physical environment of the panicky patient is used as an adjunct to reassurance. All other persons, such as relatives and attendants, are removed form the presence of the patient so that you and the patient are in a quiet office. This action reassures the patient that you do not fear the patient's loss of control, that a guard or attendant is not needed, and that you are aready to offer help.

Empathy

A patient who is working very hard with deep-seated feelings says, "I just can't stand it here in this room any longer. I want out of the room."

Question: What would be an empathic response?

Answer: Does your response recognize the feeling and show acceptance of it? The patient is restless or panicky or irritated with working this hard, with having to deal with an unpleasant experience, and with being dependent upon you for help. Thus you might respond with:
This work gets to you after a few minutes.
It's no fun dealing with these feelings and having to be dependent upon someone else for help, is it?

Empathy, as used here, helps the patient to express his/her feelings more directly, dealing with them openly and without embarrassment.

It is important to realize that an empathic response does not involve giving advice, giving reassurance, doing something about the feeling, or even saying that the feeling is or is not justified. One merely recognizes the feeling and allows and accepts the patient's expression of it.

A patient says after a week of following a diet, "I surely thought that I would be able to lose weight. I have done the best I can. I tried everything that you told me to do but nothing seems to work."

Question: Write out an empathic response to this patient.

Answer: Does your response name the patient's feeling and accept his/her having it and expressing it?

Question: Which of the following is an empathic response to this patient? What would be wrong with using the other responses?
A. This new diet came in the morning mail; let's shift over to it.
B. When you try hard and still are unable to lose weight, no one can blame you for being discouraged.
C. Don't be too impatient, give the diet a little time.
D. When you can't seem to lose weight, I can see how you would be discouraged.

Answer: A ignores the patient's feeling and gives directions or advice which would close the subject to further understanding. It also abandons the notion that the diet is good in and of itself.
B names and accepts the feelings, but it also provides an unnecessary justification for the feeling.
C is a mild reprimand to the patient for showing his/her feelings and also gives advice.
D is empathic.

A patient says, "Since I hurt my arm on the job, the company doctor saw me twice. He took some X-rays and said it was all okay. He saw me just one more time and gave me a prescription for the pain, but didn't suggest any exercises or heat treatments. I felt he wasn't doing all that he could. He wanted me to return to work and not use any of my Workmen's Compensation. He should have really done more for me."

Question: Make up a response that will empathize with the patient, but do not justify his feeling, since this may further his incapacity.

Answer: Your response might be similar to one of the following:
You felt a little unhappy with the doctor's treatment?
You felt that your arm needed more attention?
You felt that he should have done more for you?
You felt that he did not show you enough concern?

Support

Supportive responses can either enhance the patient's description of his/her illness or it can close the topic to further discussion.

A patient says, "I don't know what to do when I take the medicine and get no relief. I want to go to sleep, but the pain keeps me awake and then I just don't know what to do."

Question: Which of the following responses would lead to further discussion and which ones would close the topic?
A. It is not unusual for patients to complain of this trouble. I know how you must feel.

B. That surely is upsetting. Such a pain upsets anyone. It will be better.
C. This is the most difficult part of your treatment. It will be better.
D. Don't be upset about it, you will feel much better next week.
E. This is a difficult time. You feel that you need something more at night?

Answer: A, B, C, and D all tend to close the topic to further discussion. Think for a moment how you, as a patient, would respond to each. E, on the other hand, requests the patient to continue talking about what he/she feels is needed.

Direct reassurance, given early, tends to close a discussion. Empathy and support are just as helpful to the patient and do not tend to close the discussion. From time to time each type of response is useful.

A patient recovering from surgery says, "I have been waiting for 3 months. Will I get over this and be able to eat as I did before?" You do not know what this patient has been thinking and with what he has scared himself. You want to know what his fears are. He is asking for support. You believe that he will be able to eat as before.

Question: What is the supportive response that does not close the topic to discussion?

Answer: Compare your answer to the following:
Why do you ask?
Now what is on your mind that prompts this question?
Sounds like you have been doing a lot of thinking.

These responses are not supportive on the surface, but they show your interest in him is very supportive. A directly supportive response might be:
Yes, but you seem to be having some doubts?

CONFRONTATION

confrontation a response that points out to the patient his/her feeling, behavior, or previous statement.*
Confrontations are most effective in focusing the patient's attention upon his/her feeling, behavior, or statement. They may also let the patient know you understand what he/she said. Many times a special inflection or insinuation is made in repeating his/her statement to emphasize a part of it.

Question: Which of the following might be considered a confrontation?
A. You look unhappy.
B. When I touch here, you grimace.
C. You are saying the other professionals didn't understand how much trouble you are having?
D. Where did you say the pain is?

---

*Enelow, A. J., and Wexler, M.: Psychiatry in the practice of medicine, New York, 1966, Oxford University Press, Inc., pp. 59-60.

Answer: A, B, and C may be considered confrontations.
D merely asks for a point of information that you missed.

You learn from a patient who has intermittent joint pain that he had a bad attack last Saturday. He said that nothing happened to cause the attack. You then get him to tell you about Saturday and he says, "After about an hour of work at the office I went to the airport to pick up my father-in-law. We went to lunch and then home with the family. That afternoon we sat around and talked. I first noticed the pain at lunch." You know from previous information that his father-in-law owns the business he operates, so you want to focus on the fact that his father-in-law came to town.

Question: What is your response?

Answer: The following are several examples of confrontations:
You met your father-in-law at the airport?
Nothing happened Saturday to cause an attack but you did meet your father-in-law at the airport?
Your father-in-law came to town Saturday?

A patient tells you, in a complaining way, "The treatments you are giving me are costing too much." You sense that the patient wants you to change the treatment.

Question: What is your response?

Answer: Compare your response with the following:
You sound like you want me to change your treatment.
Too much? Is the price really a problem?
You seem to be complaining about the treatment.

A young male patient tells you, "My father feels I am taking too much medicine for this pain." As the patient tells you this, you notice his fist clenches. You wish to focus his attention on your observation.

Question: Make up a response that will confront this young man with his behavior.

Answer: Compare your response with the following:
Were you aware you clenched your fist when you spoke of your father's feeling?
You said that with a clenched fist.

REFLECTION

reflection   a response that repeats, mirrors, or echoes a portion of what the patient just said.
Although it focuses on a particular point, a reflection helps the patient to continue in his/her own style.

Question: Which of the following might be reflections?
A. And then?
B. It hurt?
C. You could not eat?
D. Nervous?

Answer: B, C, and D

A would be a reflection if the patient had said, "and then . . ." without completing the sentence. Otherwise it would be considered an open-ended question.

A patient says, "I have hurt for three weeks. Then last Saturday I noticed it all seemed to focus on a pain in my left side."

Question: Reflect this statement and focus the patient on the pain so that the patient can continue.

Answer: Did your response use the exact words the patient used? If not, you should have. Compare your response with ours:
Focus on a pain?
In your left side?
Hurt Saturday in your left side?

A patient says, "The pain was worse last night. It was really bad."

Question: Reflect this statement to the patient to learn what he means by "bad."

Answer: We would focus his attention on bad by asking:
Bad?
It was bad?
The pain was worse?

INTERPRETATION

interpretation   a confrontation that is based upon an inference rather than upon an observation.*

An interpretation usually links events or ascribes motives or feeling to the patient's reply or behavior.

Question: Which of the following might be considered to be an interpretation?
Which is a confrontation?
A. You seem to be unhappy.
B. You upset me.
C. You just clenched your fist.
D. Sounds like you do not like the assistant.
E. You reacted the same way when you lost your job.

Answer: A, D, and E are interpretations.
B and C report your unaltered observation of the patient and of your own reaction and are thus confrontations.

A patient says, "When I went into the supervisor's office this morning, this pain in my chest was really bad." You learned earlier that on a previous visit to the supervisor's office, and even as a child going to his father's study, the patient would have increased discomfort from aches and pains.

---

*Blyth, J. M., and Alter, M.: How to conduct a selection interview, Los Angeles, 1965, Sherbourne Press, p. 357.
Enelow, A. J., and Wexler, M.: Psychiatry in the practice of medicine, New York, 1966, Oxford University Press, Inc., pp. 59-60.

Question: Interpret this information to the patient, making an inference concerning the association or cause, and confront the patient with this information.

Answer: Compare your responses with the following:
Interpretation:
Sounds like seeing the supervisor now was like seeing your father when you were a child. Both make your pains worse.
Confrontation:
Just when you went in?
Into the supervisor's office?
Your pain became worse?
Just by going into the supervisor's office?

SILENCE

silence a communication, a response.

Those scientists who study communication report that *we cannot fail to communicate.* A silence can show interest or lack of interest; it can also show support or withdrawal. Most useful to the professional are the supportive silence and the interested silence.

A patient says, "I'm unhappy about the way this pain persists." You want the patient to tell you more about the feelings.

Question: How might you respond?
A. Uh huh!
B. Silence, looking at the patient's record.
C. Silence, nod "yes."
D. Silence, a relaxed shift back into your chair.
E. Silence, shift forward in your chair with increased attention.

Answer: A, C, and E would show interest and support in what the patient is saying. Your interest and support would encourage further discussion of the topic by the patient.
B is usually interpreted by patients as a withdrawal from them or a display of lack of interest or both.
D may be interpreted either as a withdrawal from the patient or as "now I am relaxed and ready to really listen."

The patient interprets your silence positively when you focus your attention on the patient and away from objects on your desk or table next to you.

Patients frequently come to the professional's office with the idea or an assumed contract that they are in the interview only to answer specific questions. To counter this belief, silence early in the interview may make the interchange much more productive and could make your job as interviewer much easier.

Interviewer: What troubles are you having?
Patient: I just don't seem to have any energy. (Pause—waiting for your next question.)

Question: How would you respond to this patient? If you use silence, describe your nonverbal behavior.

Answer: Silence, accompanied by nodding your head, looking at the patient expectantly, or shifting your body toward the patient, might be used as a response.

Silence, used too much, may be interpreted by the patient to mean that the interviewer cannot think of anything to say. The patient must feel the responsibility for breaking the silence. If he/she does not feel this responsibility, silence is usually an ineffective facilitation. Silence is frequently ineffective with young teenagers since they do not feel compelled to fill the void.

Another aspect of the use of silence may be brought out by the following dialogue:

Interviewer: When did you first notice the pain?

Patient: Let's see (pause) first I noticed the pain last August, (pause) no, it was while I was away at summer school. It was about (pause) the middle of July (pause).

Question: How would you respond to this patient, a college student?

Answer: This student is having some difficulty remembering the history of his pain and needs some time to collect his thoughts. Silence on your part can be very supportive, but silence beyond 10 seconds would not be appropriate in this situation.

Question: If, after 15 seconds, the student remained silent, how would you respond?

Answer: Compare your response with the following:
What was it like then?
Once the time of the onset of the present problem is established, the quality of the symptoms and the associated events at that time are the next logical pieces of information to obtain.

Question: If a patient were to begin crying while describing a severely frightening sensation, how would the patient react to a response of supportive, interested silence?

Answer: The patient would probably react positively, gain composure, and be able to continue the interview. Most patients feel that, somehow, the interviewer understands them and is able to accept them. Silence here shows acceptance of the act of crying.

Question: How would this crying patient react to firm reassurance that things will be better, such as, "Now that's alright, you will feel better"?

Answer: The patient might feel guilty about making you feel uncomfortable. When the professional uses active reassurance, many patients feel that they have done something wrong in crying.

Question: How would this same patient react to a specific question for information such as, "What did you do to get more comfortable?"

Answer: This type of response would usually make the patient feel weak and silly for crying and make him/her feel that crying was not accepted in this office. However, this question might be appropriate after a period of silence during which the patient regains composure. The timing of the question is all important.

Question: How would this patient react to silence accompanied by some bodily contact such as grasping the hand or placing your hand on the patient's nearest shoulder?

Answer: The patient's reaction will depend upon his/her interpretation of your behavior. Your behavior might be interpreted as being appropriate parental concern or supportive human understanding. On the other hand, it may be interpreted either as inappropriate seductiveness or as active reassurance, which would tend to block further emotional display.

TOUCH

A patient's acceptance of, and reaction to, physical contact will depend on a number of variables: how the physical contact is made, the age differential between the patient and the professional, the sex of each, and the timing of the action. The timing is important with respect to the length of the professional-client relationship and with respect to the amount of time passing after the crying begins and before the physical contact is made.

In an interview situation the point to remember is that physical contact is interpreted on the basis of cultural expectancies that are preconscious (they are unconscious but can readily be brought into consciousness). The saying "the message is in the receiver" has special significance in this situation. Your best intentioned touch may be misinterpreted. The following touch spectrum may be helpful in understanding your (sender) intentions and possible patient (receiver) interpretations:

Touch spectrum

11	10	9	8	7	6	5	4	3	2	1	0
Category			Feeling					Action			

Category	Feeling	Action
Avoidance		
0	Ignore	Withdrawal
Affection		
1	Greeting	Handshake
2	Caring	Arm on or around shoulder
3	Affection	Hug
Sensuality		
6	Skin feeding	Massage or stroking
Sexuality		
9	Feeling turned on sexually	Holding, stroking sensitive areas
10	Want to have sexual intercourse	Skin to skin intimate touch
11	Genitality	Sexual intercourse

From the above it may become evident to you that where you are on the spectrum may not be evident to the patient and can be easily misinterpreted. If you are not sure what the patient's expectancies are, it is best to follow the rule: *When there is hesitation, no manipulation.* You might find it comfortable to say, "I would like to comfort you, may I put my hand on your shoulder?" or, "Is it ok with you if I put my hand on your shoulder?" (This last statement does not clarify the level of either of you on the touch spectrum.)

summation a response of an interviewer that reviews information given by the patient.

A summation response may fulfill any one of several purposes: It demonstrates the interviewer's interest in the patient's history and it lets the patient know exactly how the interviewer understands what the patient has presented. By summation the patient's history may be clarified. One technique of summation consists of restating what the patient related, with reemphasis. Through reemphasis the interviewer can express such ideas as, "Is this what you (the patient) really intended to say?" or "I am interested in this particular aspect of what you said, let's explore this further." A summation may also be used to bridge a change of topic.

The following are examples of summation responses:

Now, as I understand you, the pain *is* worse after meals and you never have pain at night. (This response presents the interviewer's understanding and clarifies the history.)

Do I understand you to say that you have *never* had any trouble before the episode last week? (This response questions, for clarification, what the patient has said.)

Let me review. You said that just before you sit down you notice a sharp pain? (This response allows the interviewer to make sure the patient said what he/she had intended to say.)

Let's see, the first heart attack was in 1963 and the next one was in 1965? (This response focuses attention on 1965 and bridges a change of topic from 1963 to 1965.)

Question: A 27-year-old graduate student's wife, mother of two children, tells of her unhappiness. She says that after the first 6 months of their marriage she has never attained a sexual climax with her husband. During her first pregnancy her husband showed no interest in her. However, a male friend did show interest in her during the pregnancy, and she had relations with him that led to a climax. Further interviewing indicates that her husband was more interested in her between pregnancies but again lost interest in her during her second pregnancy. As far as she is concerned, relations between them at the present time are a mechanical act without feeling. She concludes her comments with, "He demands to have relations with me. Sometimes I refuse, but other times I submit and then can't wait until it is over. I put on an act so that he thinks I am enjoying it, but I don't enjoy it. If you asked him, he would probably say that I reach a climax every time. He just doesn't know." Make up a separate summation response that does each of the following:
A. Clarifies the history
B. Questions the patient's account
C. Focuses attention on one aspect of the history

Answer: As you compare your answers with ours, you may note that they all focus attention to an aspect of the history and, in part, question what the patient has just said.

A. Clarifies the history: "You mean to say that he doesn't know whether or not you have a climax?"
B. Questions the patient's account: "You say that he demands to have relations and you can't wait until it is over?" (This infers that the patient doesn't enjoy any part of the act.)
C. Focuses attention on one aspect of the history: "Let's review now; you say that you put on an act and you don't let him know how you really feel?"

CHAPTER 4

OBTAINING SPECIFIC INFORMATION

LAUNDRY-LIST QUESTION

Frequently, a patient will reply to a facilitation or an open-ended question with the question, "How do you mean?" The following exchange is an example.

Interviewer: Tell me about your pain.

Mr. Adams: It just hurts.

Interviewer: It hurts?

Mr. Adams: Yes!

Interviewer: Tell me about it.

Mr. Adams: How do you mean?

The interviewer has now used a reflection and two open-ended questions without getting a description of the pain. At this point Mr. Adams needs some support and guidance. A technique frequently used in this situation is a laundry-list question that gives the patient a number of alternative adjectives or descriptive phrases to use.

Question: Which of the following might be considered a laundry-list question?

A. Is it a burning pain?

B. Does the pain go up over your head?

C. Does the pain feel like a burn, ache, drawing, pressure, or piercing?

D. Does it come on every week, every hour, every month, or every few minutes?

Answer: C and D

Patient: This pain is worse.

Interviewer: How is that?

Patient: What do you mean?

Question: How would you phrase a laundry-list question to learn what the patient means by "worse?"

Answer: Compare your answer with the following:
Well, is it more frequent, deeper, making your whole jaw ache, keeping you awake, or what?

Question: What would be wrong with a laundry-list question such as the following:

Do you have these pains every hour, day, or week?

Answer: There are two possible errors in this question:
1. The patient is reluctant to give an answer that falls outside the range of frequencies that have been suggested. The above question sets the limits from one hour to one week. The patient may hesitate to answer that the pains occur every 20 minutes.
2. Since the order of frequency given in the question falls into a logical sequence, it usually gives some hint to the patient of what you expect the answer to be. Many times it is the voice inflection that gives away the expected answer.

To avoid suggesting the answer, the rule in formulating a laundry-list question is to scramble the logical sequence of items and to give limits beyond those which any patient would be expected to answer.

Question: If a patient were having attacks of pain and you wanted to know how frequent they were, how would you phrase a laundry-list question? (Usual frequency is from one attack per day to one every 2 to 3 days.)

Answer: Compare your answer to the following, which limits but illustrates the technique:

Do you have attacks once a week, once an hour, once a month, once every 5 minutes, or once a year?

A modification of the laundry-list question can be used to draw out a patient to tell you more. When the list is limited to two items, both of which are absurd, the patient must then clarify his position.

Question: Which of the following examples would draw out the patient?
A. Is your pain just barely annoying or has it stopped you from working?
B. I don't understand, does your pain make you vomit or can you ignore it and continue what you are doing?

Answer: Both. A pain is more than annoying if the patient is coming to the office about it, and most pains do not cause one to stop working or cause one to vomit.

DIRECT QUESTION

direct question A response that asks for a specific bit of information. A direct question can usually be answered in one word or a brief phrase.*

In the opening dialogue Mr. Adams was not able to give us a description of the pain with the aid of open-ended questions and facilitations.

Question: What would be wrong with using one of the following questions after Mr. Adams mentioned his pain?

---

*Enelow, A. J., and Wexler, M.: Psychiatry in the practice of medicine, New York, 1966, Oxford University Press, Inc., p. 57.

A. Did it keep you awake at night?
B. Is it a throbbing pain?
C. Does the pain seem to be in one spot?

Answer: Some of the faults with these questions are as follows:

1. You would be asking for a "yes" or "no" from the patient, either of which will yield little information.
2. You would be giving the patient some information as to what you thought the pain might be like or (as he would see it) what the pain *should* be like.
3. From these questions you would get confirmation or denial of your own concept of what the patient's pain is like, not his candid description.
4. You would encourage an authoritarian-submissive or parent-child relationship with the patient.
5. The burden of interpreting the meaning of the questions is placed upon the patient. Since you are not sure what his interpretation is, you will not be sure what his answer means.

Direct questions that can be answered with one word add little information to what you already have about the patient. On the other hand, they may provide that crucial bit of information that is diagnostic.

Question: Which of the following questions would result in more information?

A. Is it a burning pain?
B. What is the pain like?
C. What seems to aggravate your pain?
D. Does the pain get worse when you eat?

Answer: B and C
A and D yield a very specific bit of information that could be answered by a "yes" or "no."

We do not wish to advocate avoiding all questions with one-word answers. At times such questions are the most appropriate, but these times are few. After a patient has given you a description of his pain that fits the symptoms of a particular ailment (i. e., abscess) you need to ask specific questions related to the ailment.

Question: Which of the following would you ask?

A. What have you noticed in the area of the pain?
B. Have you had any pus from the area of the pain?
C. What changes have you noticed in the area of the pain?

Answer: B will give you the information you desire and will save valuable interview time. The direct question can also be used to focus a rambling patient on the topic of concern.

PROBING

In telling of their symptoms, patients do not give you all the details you need. Once they have told you about a phase of the illness, it may be necessary to probe for more specific information.

Question: Which of the following would probe for more detailed information?

A. And then?
B. What else did you notice at the time?
C. Mm hmmmm.

Answer: A and B
C would allow the patient to change the subject or proceed in any direction.

A patient has told you that she sometimes has pain in her stomach after lunch. It lasts about half an hour.

Question: You want to know if there are specific foods associated with the pain. Which of the following would you ask to obtain this information?
A. What do you notice about the days when you have the pain?
B. Is there something different about the consistency or hardness of the food you eat on the days you have pain?
C. Do you avoid certain foods to prevent pain?
D. Do you eat the same thing every day at lunch?
E. Tell me more about that.

Answer: B, C, and D
A and E wander too far from the information that you want.

A patient tells you about an abdominal pain that is worse in the morning and after a day in which he was tense and smoked more than usual. He tells you of its frequency, persistence, and about the discomfort associated with it. You observe a splinting of his side. You want to know whether the patient has any swelling or color change in the area of his side.

Question: Phrase a probing question that does not give away the answer or frighten the patient.

Answer: Compare your answer with the following:
What does your side look like?
What changes have you noticed in your side?
Are there any changes in the skin on your side?

Before you get the final answer on whether the patient has a swelling or color change, you may have to follow up these questions with an additional question such as: "Are there any color changes in the skin of your side?"

CHANGE OF TOPIC

An interview is created from a number of merging topics. The professional guides and directs the selection of topics through many of the techniques discussed earlier and by deliberately changing (or preventing the patient from changing) the topic.

The patient has given you a very complete description of his present symptoms of a possible genetic defect. You wish to learn if anyone in his family has had similar symptoms. You want to change the topic and focus on his family.

Question: Which of the following would you ask?
A. Does anyone in your family have similar symptoms?
B. Do you know anyone with similar problems?

27

C. I would like to know about your family. Has anyone in your family had similar symptoms?

Answer: A implies that the symptoms are caused by something in the family.

B is too open-ended, since the patient is free to talk about friends and co-workers. Also, it does not prepare the patient for a change in topic.

C is preferred because it gives the patient a reason for the question. He is not left to guess why you changed the subject. From C he may well infer that you are just being thorough and avoiding using diagnostic terms.

When you change the subject, it is good practice to let the patient know why; otherwise, his/her inferences may get in the way of treatment. If there is no logical bridge from one topic to the next, say so. Be honest with the patient. If there is a logical bridge, give it. By your concerned frankness and honesty, you will encourage the patient to be frank and honest with you.

Question: What is wrong with this exchange?
Patient: Well, I guess that's the entire story of my case of venereal sores in my mouth. I should have come in sooner. (Pause.)
Interviewer: How is your mother's health?

Answer: Since the interviewer did not present a logical association, the patient might well reply, "Now what kind of a question is that? My mother doesn't have anything to do with my illness."

Question: How could the interviewer have asked the question to obtain the needed information as a logical sequence?

Answer: Compare your answer to the following:
That may be true but we can still help you. Now let me review the health of your family. How is your mother's health?
That may be true but we can still help you. Now let me get some medical history of your family. How is your mother's health?

Interviewer: What seems to be the trouble?
Patient: I have had this pain for some time now. It is getting worse. Last night I hardly slept at all because of the discomfort.
Interviewer: What is it like?
Patient: It feels like it is down here in the middle of my arm. Then my shoulder gets sore and I just can't get comfortable. All of this makes my arm worse and it begins to throb.

Question: You want to focus on the pain in the arm and come back to the soreness in the shoulder later. What is your response?

Answer: Does your answer let the patient know that you plan to come back to the sore shoulder? Compare your response with the following:
I need more information about the pain first and then we can come back to your sore shoulder. You mentioned that you have had the pain for some time. (Pause and wait for the patient to say more about it.)

CHAPTER 5

SPECIFIC INTERVIEW PROBLEMS

QUESTIONS THAT ANTAGONIZE

"According to your record you have not lost any weight. Why do you keep eating so much?"

Question: What is wrong with this question?

Answer: This question antagonizes the patient, accuses him/her of wrong-doing, and tends to put the patient on the defensive. If you put a patient on the defensive, he/she will probably say very little and is not encouraged to cooperate with you and tell the truth.

Question: If the patient were at ease with you, he/she would speak

_____ and you would obtain a much more reliable history.

Answer: freely

In each of the following pairs of words there is an emotionally neutral and an emotionally charged word.

Question: Select the emotionally neutral word from each pair.
  A. Cancer—Growth
  B. Unsatisfactory—Bad
  C. Upset—Mad
  D. Blood colored—Reddish
  E. Doesn't care—Casual
  F. Inform—Complain
  G. Order—Ask
  H. Yellow—Jaundiced

Answer: A. Growth
  B. Unsatisfactory
  C. Upset
  D. Reddish
  E. Casual
  F. Inform
  G. Ask
  H. Yellow

Question: Select the question in each pair that is less provoking of defensiveness.

A. Why did you stop eating?
B. What was it that made eating solid foods impossible?

C. Did you think you had a growth?
D. Did you think you had a cancer?

E. That must have made you made.
F. That must have upset you.

G. Did you give in to the pain?
H. Did the pain force you to stop what you were doing?

I. How long have you treated this yourself before coming in?
J. How long have you suffered with this?

Answer: B, C, F, H, and J.

Question: Rephrase the following so that the emotionally loaded connotation, which may antagonize, is taken out:

A. Did you follow my directions in taking the medicine?
B. Why did you quit working?
C. Why did you wait until tonight to see about this?
D. Now just tell me what you noticed about the pain in your arm without all of the other information.

Answer: Compare your responses with the following:

A. How are you taking your medicine now?
B. What caused you to stop working?
C. Were you able to see about this earlier?
D. Let's just focus on the pain in your arm so that I can understand what you are experiencing.

The real world is rarely divided into black and white, all or nothing. It is made up of shades or degrees of a quality, sensation, or feeling. A professional's questions need to take this into account and ask for the degree of a sensation rather than a choice between the extremes. More information will come forth if sought in terms of degrees rather than absolutes.

Question: Choose the question below that will obtain more information.

A. Do you have difficulty eating?
B. What foods are you able to eat?

Answer: B
To A that patient may reply with "yes" or "no" and feel no pressure to say more. In reality the patient may be having some trouble chewing solids, but from your question he may not think that it is enough difficulty to justify a "yes" reply. In this situation the patient decides where to draw the line between "no difficulty" and "difficulty" and answers accordingly. With B you obtain the information from the patient and then you decide whether the patient's difficulties fit into your category of "no difficulty" or "difficulty." From B you obtain more information and take responsibility for judging the significance of the patient's experience rather than having the patient make these judgments.

Question: Select the question in each pair that obtains more precise information and underscore the phrase that makes it so:

    A. Is is possible that you were at fault when you were injured?

    B. Is it possible that you were partially at fault when you were injured?

    C. Have you had sore throats?

    D. Have you had more than one sore throat per year?

    E. Do you have headaches that are not relieved by aspirin?

    F. Do you have headaches?

Answer: B. partially

    D. more than one sore throat per year

    E. that are not relieved by aspirin

We have considered questions that may antagonize a patient because they accuse him/her of doing wrong or because they scare the patient with an emotionally loaded word. We have also considered questions that make the patient decide whether or not the degree of a quality is sufficient in his/her experience to justify a "yes" answer. Finally, we have considered questions that vary in the degree of specificity in which they direct the patient to answer. In regard to the last pairs of questions presented, the broader, less specific question is usually more appropriate when a topic is being opened, whereas the more specific question is usually more appropriate in the later discussion of a topic. When you are opening a topic your intent is to gather as much data as possible as quickly as possible. Thus, general questions and facilitations are used. Later in the discussion, when you are ready to wrap up the topic and pull in missing bits of information, more specific questions are more appropriate.

The key point is that you must be in charge and conscious of what you are doing. With practice you can precisely direct an interview in its gentleness, lack of antagonism, degree of specificity, and degree of comfort for the patient.

There are times when the situation warrants the risk and your rapport is sufficient to allow you to provoke, confront aggressively, and be blunt with the patient. These procedures are sometimes indicated to move the passive or dependent patient, to convince the patient that he/she needs to modify behavior, or to convince the patient that you care enough to risk losing his/her good feelings toward you or to risk losing him/her as a patient. Just know what you are doing, why you are doing it, and when you want to be warm, friendly, and compassionate and when you want to be difficult, confrontive, and direct. There are times when each style is appropriate and constructive for patient growth and patient acceptance of increased responsibility.

Introductory and softening phrases are useful when obtaining the social and personal information from a patient.

Question: Modify the following questions to make them more acceptable to a patient:

    A. Did the situation anger you?

    B. Was it your fault that she was upset with you?

    C. Were you unhappy on the job?

    D. Do you get irritated with people who do not follow your directions?

Answer: Compare your answers with the following:
- A. Would you say that the situation tended to anger you?
- B. Do you feel that it was partially your fault that she was upset with you?
- C. Is it possible that you were unhappy on the job?
- D. Would you be willing to say that people who do not follow your directions annoy you?

"YES" AND "NO" ANSWERS

With some patients there is a danger in using questions requiring "yes" and "no" answers. The patient's answer may be more dependent on the immediate milieu than on the facts.

When a question is answered with a "yes," you cannot be sure what the "yes" means. Is it given to please you, to give you what the patient thinks you want to hear, to avoid discussing an area that the patient wants to avoid, or is it a factual response?

The following questions might be answered with "yes" for any of the above reasons.
1. Have you been able to take the medicine?
2. You saw a doctor about that trouble 3 years ago?
3. Are you getting along all right with your job now?
4. Are you able to stay on the diet?

When a question can be answered with a "no," the same situation arises as with the questions that can be answered with a "yes."

Question: The patient may just wish to disagree, wish to _____,

wish to _____ discussing the topic, or wish to give

a _____ response.

Answer: please, avoid, factual

Several examples of questions that will yield "no" answers of unknown meaning are as follows:
- A. Have you had any trouble with your ears?
- B. Do you take sedatives frequently?
- C. Did you have trouble with the false teeth?
- D. Have you been sick before?
- E. Have you had sick headaches?
- F. Do you eat excessively?
- G. Do you kick your dog?
- H. Do you scream at your children?

"WHY" QUESTIONS

Question: What is wrong with a question such as: "Why did you take that medicine?" or "Why did you leave work?" or "Why did you get a divorce?"

Answer: These questions call on the patient to account for his/her behavior. Since much of the patient's behavior may be unconscious or related to reasons that are not socially acceptable, the patient may be antagonized by the inference in the question. The patient may feel that such a question finds fault with him/her and may thus become irritated or annoyed. It is difficult to begin a question with "why" and avoid the overtones of accusation. In addition, "why" questions come from a whining position on the part of the person asking the question. The whining position may be described as a position of helplessness, pleading, or angry frustration. See if these adjectives describe your feelings the next time you find yourself asking "why" questions.

Question: What is wrong with questions such as: "Why did you have a headache Saturday afternoon?" or "Why were you so tense this morning?"

Answer: If the patient knew why he/she felt the way he/she did, the patient would understand the illness and might not need your services. In addition, the patient's usual response to one of these questions will be a rationalization.

The answer to a "why" question is a "because." Since we are not always capable of understanding our own behavior, the "because" answer is the most socially acceptable answer we can come up with. It is an alibi, an excuse, or in professional terms, a rationalization. Rationalizations are of interest to some but are little or no value in the professional interview or interaction.

An alternative to asking "why?" is to make an honest statement to the patient such as, "I am not clear . . ." or "I do not understand the situation. Tell me more how you see it." Such responses do not irritate or antagonize the patient. They show interest and are supportive. They may produce a rationalization but the patient generally does not feel as defensive as he/she would with a direct, whining "why" question.

SUGGESTIVE QUESTIONS

Interviewer: When you discussed your problem, your breathing was a little rapid. Were you at ease or were you a little nervous at the time?

Patient: I was a little nervous.

Question: What was wrong with the interviewer's question?

Answer: The interviewer gave the patient the answer as well as the question. To avoid this error the interviewer could have asked, "What was the situation when you discussed your problem?" The interviewer could then later have asked, "Were you at ease then?"

To varying degrees both the experienced interviewer and the novice ask questions that suggest the answers.

Question: Rephrase the following questions so that they do not suggest the answers:
A. Has the pain gone to the top of your head?
B. Is the pain worse when eating?
C. Some patients report nausea with this medicine. Does it affect you in this way?
D. May I assume that you have taken the medicine as directed?
E. Before taking the medicine do you always try to relieve the pain by relaxing?

Answer: Compare your rephrased questions with the following:
A. Is the pain only around your ear or do you notice it elsewhere?
B. What is the pain like after a big meal?
C. Do you have any complaints about the medicine?
D. How are you taking the medicine now?
E. What do you do to relieve the pain?

One way to test a question as to whether or not it is a give-away is to see if you can anticipate the answer.

Question: In which of the following can you anticipate the answer?
A. You take the medicine after every meal don't you?
B. Are you able to take the medicine after every meal?

Answer: A
B gives the patient an acceptable out for not following the medication directions to the letter. The patient might say that he/she is unable to take the medicine at work.

You are interviewing a patient who has been injured on the job. You want to know whether or not the pain in his back goes into his neck.

Question: Rephrase the following question to remove the suggestion that the pain might be expected to go into the patient's neck: "Does the pain ever shoot into your neck?"

Answer: Is the pain only in your back?
Do you notice the pain anywhere else?

PATIENT QUESTIONS

Patients ask questions for many different reasons. When a patient asks a question during data gathering, the patient is asking rarely for information. These questions are usually designed for other reasons. The reason for the question is not always clear.

Question: How would you respond to, "Are you married? Do you have any children?"
A. If the patient seemed to be asking a simple question for information.
B. If the patient seemed to be trying to manipulate the professional relationship.

Answer: A. A simple, direct, honest reply of "yes" or "no" would be appropriate. We assume that the patient wishes to know you as a real person rather than as an idealized role image. If you were correct in your assumption that the patient was just asking for information, the topic will change.
B. "Why do you ask?" if done noncombatively is always a safe answer. We assume in this case that the patient is asking the question to modify the professional relationship toward one that is closer, informal, and social. Should you respond "yes," you invite a more personal question such as, "Is your wife/ husband happy?" or "Does your husband/wife feel lucky to have you?" These questions may lead to a nonprofessional relationship problem. Prevent this problem before it occurs.

The rule is to answer a patient's personal questions honestly and directly *only* when you understand clearly why they are asked and when you are confident that your reply will further the maintenance of a comfortable professional relationship.

Question: How would you respond to questions such as: "Are you a Democrat?" or "Are you a Baptist?" or "Are you Jewish?"

Answer: These questions are generally inappropriate for a patient to ask. Your response should indicate that discussion of these topics does not contribute to the patient's care. Compare your answers to the following:

It is interesting that you ask that, but what I need to know is . . .

Why do you ask?

I don't understand how that will make a difference in my helping you.

Question: If a patient replies, "Oh, I was just wondering how you were going to vote," how would you respond?

Answer: Compare your response with the following:

I don't see how that information will help us get your problem solved.

Question: Knowing that the patient has cancer, how would you respond to, "Do I have cancer?"

Answer: "Cancer" is a word that is emotionally loaded and that has, medically speaking, lost its dictionary meaning. Thus, you cannot answer the question with a simple sentence. As illustrated in the drawing, what the patient has in his head when he thinks about the word "cancer" may be quite different from what the professional has in his head when he thinks about the word "cancer"

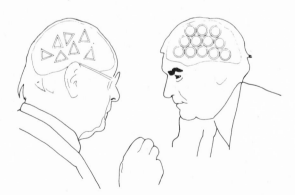

You must answer the question by discussing for 5 to 10 minutes what the patient has been thinking about and what he really wants to know. An answer such as the following might initiate this discussion: "I don't know what you mean by "cancer," but maybe we can discuss exactly what you do have. Let's start with what you have been thinking about and what questions you have."

The response, "Why do you ask?" may work very well in this situation, but it does have a gently discouraging quality to it and may offend a sensitive patient, when that is not your intention.

Question: How would you respond to "Should I continue to practice both exercises?"
A. If the patient were asking a simple question for information.
B. If the patient were complaining about having to do so many exercises.

Answer: A. "Yes" or "no." There are situations and questions to which direct answers are indicated. Nevertheless giving direct answers in professional interviews is the exception, not the rule.
B. "What is your feeling about the exercises?" or "Do you want to continue doing both exercises?" Since the patient decides at home whether or not to do the exercise, bringing his/her feelings about the exercises out into the open may make the difference between successful and unsuccessful management of the patient.

The reason many patients ask a question is not to obtain an answer but rather to direct discussion to the topic introduced by the question, to avoid the current topic, or to direct and take more control of the interaction. Rarely does the initial question cover what the patient really wants to know. As in the question about cancer, the patient wants to know about specifics of what he/she can expect rather than the general information which would have been obtained by a "yes" or "no" answer.

INFORMING ABOUT ILLNESS

Question: You have just received the evaluation confirming that a patient under your care has a psychologic illness. How will you inform the patient or a relative of the illness?

Answer: The following is one approach: "How are you?" Obtain the patient's reply. Follow up the patient's reply by asking, "What is your understanding of what is wrong with you?" It is best to start with what the patient knows about the illness, since you may not have a clear idea of what the patient knows or fears about the illness.

Question: After learning of the patient's concept of the illness, how will you advise him/her of the true nature of the illness?

Answer: One way is to give the patient the medical diagnosis and then interpret it. For example, you might say, "Mr. Lewis, we have received the report from the psychologist on his evaluation. The diagnosis is an acute toxic reaction. What do you know about this disease?"

Question: Mr. Lewis replies, "I never heard of that before." Now what will you say to him?

Answer: You might ask, "What questions do you have about it?" It is best to begin with information that the patient wants to know rather than with information that the patient does not want, cannot handle intellectually or emotionally, or will not hear for a variety of reasons. A patient's concern is usually whether or not he/she will recover, be able to return to work, have pain, or will need special treatment. If surgery is needed, the patient wants to know if it will be disfiguring.

A part of helping the patient learn about his/her illness is to get the patient to answer his/her own questions by asking, "What do you think?" and then correcting the answers. The patient may ask specific questions to which it is best to answer as honestly as you can, keeping in mind that you never want to destroy the patient's defenses. Remember, you are helping the patient learn about the disease, you are not showing off how much you know. What the patient ends up knowing is what is important, not how good you looked in the process. You want to let the patient know that regardless of what he/she is to go through, you will be supportive.

Remember, the most important part of a message is that part heard by the receiver. In this situation you are imparting information to the patient. The most important part of the process is learning what the patient hears.

Question: After you have answered the patient's questions and discussed the patient's illness, what should you say before you close the conversation?

Answer: Compare your answer to the following:
I'm concerned that we have a common understanding of your situation. Let's review how you see it now.
You will be amazed how frequently the patient's understanding is in error. If possible, you should correct the patient's misconceptions. This may not be possible when the patient has some personal need to misunderstand, such as a need to deny any imperfection in him/herself. When such a block to understanding occurs, note it and leave the resolution for a time when the patient is more receptive.

Question: How might you close the discussion?

Answer: Compare your answer to the following:
You may have further questions by your next visit. If so, please ask them. I will see you again at your next appointment and we will discuss your questions at that time.

In caring for a patient with an illness that will persist for some time or for a patient who will need further therapy, it is important to encourage the patient to ask any questions. This will help the patient to avoid worry. The patient who does not ask questions to clarify ideas may develop a delusion about what is going on in his/her body. Such a delusion may prevent or interfere with treatment.

After news of a fatal illness, the patient will obviously be anxious and have many worrisome thoughts about what the future holds. The anxious patient often cannot clearly understand instructions about control of pain or taking of medications. It is a good procedure to check out what the patient heard you say, what he/she understands, and how he/she will handle bleeding, pain, or other predictable occurrences. The process of giving instructions is similar to the process of informing the patient of a serious illness. Use the same follow-through and checking techniques, and you will have fewer calls outside of office hours.

In summary, the steps for informing a patient or a patient's relative of an illness are:

1. Find out what the patient or relative thinks or knows about the illness.
2. Find out what the patient or relative wants to know about the illness.
3. Give honest answers to the questions in such a way that you leave the patient or relative with a realistic hope.
4. Before you close the conversation, determine the patient's or relative's understanding of what you have discussed.
5. Leave the communication channel open so that the patient or relative can ask further questions.

For the specific situation of having to inform a patient of a fatal illness, we suggest that you review in chapters 3 and 4 *Communication With The Fatally Ill* by Adriaan Verwoerdt.*

INTERVIEWING TRAPS

There are many common traps into which the beginning, and even at times the experienced, interviewer falls. Some of these traps are covered in earlier discussions of specific techniques to be used in conducting the interview.

The question that can be answered with a "yes" or "no" is fraught with miscommunications. Reasons for the patient responding with a "yes" or "no" may range from giving factual information to wanting to please or displease you. The patient may even be trying to avoid further discussion of the topic or hasten the end of the interview.

Suggestive questions give the patient the answer to the question or at least let the patient know the answer that you are seeking. With the patient who has a need to please others, the answer will probably be what you expected to hear.

Multiple questions have one specific use and many difficulties. The one specific use is to encourage a quiet patient to take responsibility and talk more freely. By asking multiple questions, the patient (if he/she can remember all of the questions) is encouraged to start talking and to continue talking until all of the questions are answered. This is used to avoid short answers from the patient. When it works it can be very effective; however, the multiple question approach often confuses the patient, who may feel rushed, put down, confused, or pushed. If any of these feelings are present, the patient is unlikely to give meaningful information.

Silence that occurs without clear direction or meaning to the patient has been referred to as "stumped silence." In stumped silence uncertainty

---

*Verwoerdt, A.: Communication with the fatally ill, Springfield, Ill. 1966, Charles C Thomas, Publisher.

prevails. It appears that you, the interviewer, are confused or lost and are not sure what to do next. The patient is also lost and does not know what is expected. The situation is awkward for both of you. It is better to be more specific and say, "I'm not sure that I understand," rather than to stay silent and let the patient wonder what is going on. It also helps to control your own feelings and reactions so that you can identify and verbalize them. We can always adjust better to the known than to the unknown. The patient will be much more likely to adjust to the uncertainty if you can talk about it than if he/she is left with suspicions and uncertainties.

Another interviewing trap is the hasty reassurance. There is almost nothing more effective for closing a topic to discussion than to jump in with "I'm sure it will be all right." Hasty reassurance always closes the topic to discussion. When gathering data, this is the last thing you want to happen. When you need more data, reassurance will block your attempts. It is much more reassuring to be able to talk about a difficult problem than it is to have someone offer you a reassuring comment.

When the process of data-gathering produces defensiveness in the patient or in the interviewer, the effectiveness of the interview suffers. Defensiveness is usually a by-product of criticism, which is experienced as embarrassment, discomfort, shame, or rejection. Remember, it is not your job to be a judge. It is your job to understand and help the person attain his/her goals for him/herself. It is your job to let the patient be aware of alternate goals, and it is the patient's job to select which goal he/she wishes to move toward.

A common trap in informing a patient about a procedure, a treatment, or how to take medications is to assume that the patient understands what you said in the same way you understood it when you explained it. If the patient does not understand it the same way, the fault may not be in an inadequate explanation, but in not checking out how the communication was received and understood. Occasionally, the meaning of your words is quite different from the patient's understanding of them. The rule is to constantly check what is being heard and understood. Occasionally, nonverbal clues will alert you that the patient must have heard something that you did not intend.

Closely allied to the patient's understanding of your words is the trap of using jargon. When professional jargon is used, the patient may feel put down, misunderstand what you say, and be very confused. We are so accustomed to jargon that we are not aware of its use until we notice a patient's confusion. This confusion will sometimes be made evident by a question indicating that the patient's understands far less than we realized or by a patient just failing to follow our treatment program. When the patient fails to follow our plans for treatment, our first reaction should be that the patient honestly understood the treatment plan as something different from what we intended. Excessive jargon is a trap to avoid.

INTERRUPTION OF THE INTERVIEW

Question: How would you feel, as a patient, if you were being interviewed and the interviewer accepted a nonemergency telephone call?

Answer: Most patients resent the intrusion. They may feel a lack of interest by the interviewer, an uneasiness to be eavesdropping on the conversation, and irritation that their appointment time is being used for someone else. In addition, the flow of the interview is interrupted and the total situation—made up of thoughts, associations, feelings, and interaction—can never be recreated. It is lost forever.

Physicians have equated surgical procedures with interviews when considering interruptions. The surgeon allows interruptions only during minor procedures involving problems of little depth. Similarly, only in minor interviews with little depth of feeling or content are interruptions permitted.

Question: The nurse (on the service where you have just transferred a patient) calls to give you a report about the patient. You have been interviewing a new patient for 5 minutes. What response should your secretary make to the nurse?

Answer: _____ (your name) is seeing a patient, may I have him/her call you?

Question: Dr. W. calls to refer a patient to you. You have been interviewing a new patient for 5 minutes. What response should your secretary make to Dr. W.?

Answer: _____ (your name) is with a patient just now. Is there something I may do for you, or may I have him/her call you when he/she finishes?
You may feel that this reply to a physician is too blunt, but he/she must respect you and the importance of your interactions with patients. He/she would not expect you to answer the telephone while you are doing surgery with several assistants helping, so why should you be expected to answer the telephone while performing an equally difficult technique all by yourself—the interview. In some settings it is the custom for a physician to stop what he/she is doing and receive a call from another physician. When this is the case, the secretary may reply, "Is there something I can do for you now, or do you need to speak with the doctor?"

Question: There are times when the interview needs to be interrupted or when you must leave the interview. An example might be that your son just broke his leg at school and the school nurse wants you to tell her what to do. What would you say to your patient?

Answer: "Excuse me a moment." You leave, take the call on another telephone, return to the patient and say, "My son has been in an accident. I am sorry but we will have to complete this interview later. Can you wait for an hour or would you prefer another appointment?" Your approach must be honest and show concern for the patient's inconvenience.

CHAPTER 6

CLOSING THE INTERVIEW

The constructive rapport established during the interview can be destroyed by an inappropriate closing. The time at which the interview is concluded is governed by the clock. The limitations of schedule make it difficult for both the interviewer and the patient to plan their interactions so that the natural conclusion arrives when the hands of the clock reach the magic point. Even so, it is important for both the patient and the interviewer to feel that the visit has come to a natural conclusion.

The interview is closed with the same concern and thoughtfulness with which it is opened. The interviewer's opening statement sets the tone of the relationship and the direction of the interview. The closing interaction solidifies the relationship and sets the stage for the management of the problem. Several closing techniques are available to the interviewer. One is to ask the patient if he/she has any questions. The response is not meant to open a new topic, but rather to ask if there is unfinished business related to the earlier discussion. Along with this question, the more experienced interviewer will use nonverbal indications that the interview is about to be concluded. For example, he/she may look at his/her watch, may shift to a position as though ready to get up, or, if notes are taken, put the pen aside. These non-verbal signals tell the patient, "We are about to conclude this interview."

Closing an interview includes three steps—a final statement by the interviewer, a prescription for action, and the physical parting.

The *final statement* is a succinct survey of what the interviewer has learned from the interview. It is a summary. It contains information to which the interviewer and patient have already agreed. It is not controversial. The final statement is positive rather than negative. Critical comments or an unfavorable prognosis are avoided.

The *prescription for action* gives the patient a constructive plan. There is a distinction between a prescription for action and the giving of advice. A prescription for action should be based upon medical knowledge. Advice is often based upon little more than a hunch or a personal feeling. After all, why should a patient pay for advice when he/she can obtain it from anyone, anywhere, without expense. The prescription for action is derived from the interviewer's expertise and is not available from just anyone, anywhere.

The *physical parting* may be the most awkward and the most difficult part of an interview, for both the patient and the interviewer. However, the parting is but a natural conclusion to the mutually successful experience if the patient's anticipated needs have been met. The physical parting is initiated when the interviewer rises and opens the office door for the patient. Since the patient may have many concerns at this moment, it is important that the interviewer note whether or not the patient has all of his/her belongings. The interviewer's final remark may be either a reminder that he/she will look forward to seeing the patient at the next scheduled appointment or (if this is the last visit) a brief wish for good health or success.

Question: After a diagnostic interview and examination of a middle-aged insurance salesman, Mr. Baker, who has severe, episodic pain in his head, you conclude that he needs immediate hospitalization. Make up comments to terminate the visit.

Answer: *Final statement:*
Mr. Baker, my evaluation indicates that you need further diagnostic studies and relief from this pain.
Prescription for action:
As we agreed, you should be hospitalized immediately for some X-rays and rest. (Pause and await any reaction from the patient.)
Have you any questions? (answer any questions he may have.)
Physical parting:
If you need to call anyone before going to the hospital, my secretary will be happy to place the calls for you. I will see you at the hospital in a few hours. (Interviewer exits and summons his/her assistant.)

REFERRING A PATIENT

Referral to a physician or to an allied health professional can be an awkward interaction between the interviewer and the patient. The referring professional may have negative feelings about the referral. He/she may experience feelings of guilt related to a belief that he/she should know more, be perfect, or not need the help of another professional; feelings of sadness from the perception that he/she is losing a patient; feelings of frustration at being unable to meet the patient's needs; feelings of anger because the patient failed to respond to treatment; or feelings of resentment toward the patient because in some way the patient turns him/her off. Recognition of these feelings by the interviewer allows him/her to be in conscious control of them so that they have minimal effect on the referral.

Question: How should you proceed in referring a patient to another health professional? What steps should be included in the discussion with the patient about the referral to another health professional?

Answer: In the discussion with the patient the following points should be included:
1. Review your specific findings that indicate the need for the referral.
2. Take the responsibility for making the referral.

3. Describe what the patient may expect from the other professional, including cost.
4. Say what you expect from the other professional.
5. Seek the patient's acceptance of the plan.

Because of the interviewer's feelings, one of the more difficult referrals to make is to a psychiatrist. Note the preferred steps in the following example of a referral to a psychiatrist.

"*(Step 1)* Mrs. Arnold, because of your headaches, your loss of sleep, your tension, and your difficulties with your daughter, *(Step 2)* I want the assistance of Dr. K., a psychiatrist. I believe he can help us better understand what is going on and help plan your treatment. *(Step 3)* When you see Dr. K. he will talk with you probably for 45 or 50 minutes and may have one of his assistants give you some psychologic tests. His usual fee is $XX.00 per hour and testing costs vary from $YY.00 to $ZZ.00, depending upon how much testing is necessary. Dr. K. may also want to talk with your daughter and husband. *(Step 4)* After his evaluation, he will discuss his understanding of you and your problem with me and we will decide together how to best care for you. *(Step 5)* Will you agree to this referral?"

Question: What is wrong with the following referral statement?
Mrs. Arnold, from my examination I don't find anything wrong with you. I believe you should see a psychiatrist.

Answer: Mrs. Arnold may well reply, "If there is nothing wrong, why should I see a psychiatrist?" This referral is based on underlying assumptions, namely (1) if there were something organically wrong with Mrs. Arnold, the interviewer could find it, and (2) if there is no organic cause for the complaints, it must be emotional. Since medical science is not perfect, the first assumption is false. Since emotional and organic illnesses usually occur together, the second assumption is also false. *Ruling out one cause of illness does not make a positive diagnosis of another cause of the illness.*

A patient referred on the basis of the previous example goes to the psychiatrist without knowing why he/she is there. Such patient-psychiatrist interactions are initially inefficient because the contract between the patient and the psychiatrist is not clear. In fact, the referral confusion may not be able to be overcome and the consultation may be of little or no help to the patient.

Question: Make up a referral for a patient seen in the emergency room with abdominal pain. The examination reveals rebound tenderness, absent bowel sounds, and fever. You feel that a surgical consultation should be obtained on the basis of your findings.

Answer: Mrs. Arnold, because of your pain, fever, and my findings on examination of your abdomen, I want to have a surgeon see you and discuss with us the best way to help you. He will want to talk with you and reexamine you. I don't yet know whether or not you will have to stay in the hospital. Does this plan meet with your approval?

43

Question: The contract between the referring health professional and the specialist needs consideration. What does the referring health professional expect and want from the referral? What does the specialist expect and want from the consultation? At times the expectations are not in harmony. What is the problem when a specialist is accused of "patient stealing"?

Answer: The referring health professional is referring the patient for a consultation regarding diagnosis or management and the specialist believes the referring physician is sending the patient to him/her for treatment. Had the referral contract between the two been clarified, the angry feelings associated with the label "patient stealing" would not have occurred.

PART TWO

EXTENDING INTERVIEW TECHNIQUES

CHAPTER 7

MENTAL STATUS EXAMINATION

The mental status examination is part of every human interaction. When we make contact with another human being, we quickly size up where the other person is emotionally and intellectually. Most of the time this sizing-up is done preconsciously, or at least out of awareness, unless the other person does not respond to us as we expect. When the other person does not respond as expected, we wonder what is "wrong" with him/her. This sizing-up of the other person has been organized into the mental status examination. Different authors organize the information in different ways and all include information from the following topics: appearance, affect, anxiety, thinking, sensorium, and behavior. Once accurate and complete information about a person is organized into these six topics, the psychiatric diagnosis of the person's present state of functioning follows.*

APPEARANCE

The appearance of the person being interviewed is described in terms of clothing, jewelry, hair style, make-up, hygiene, skin color and texture, muscle tone, posture, gestures, facial expressions, respiration rate and depth, neck veins, scars, and amount of movement. The description of the person is that which could be recorded by a color motion picture. An interviewer is frequently judged (can be quickly assessed) as to his/her quality by how well he/she is able to describe the person that was just interviewed. We communicate much about ourselves nonverbally. A good interviewer learns to read the person by his/her appearance.

AFFECT

By affect is meant the person's feeling tone or pain-pleasure accompaniment of an idea that is experienced by the person from moment to moment. An affect is distinguished from an emotion, which is the bodily or physiologic expression of the feeling tone or affect (for example, laughing, sighing, flushing, or crying). Mood refers to a sustained or dominant affective state over a period of time.

---

*See Froelich, R. E., and Froelich, R. W.: From mental status to diagnosis, Missouri Medicine, May 1964, pp. 355-357.

The affect of the other person is described as some point on the continuum from severely withdrawn and depressed at one extreme through normal neutral feelings to the high of a manic elation. In the last few years the street people have coined many new words to describe the various states of affect from the lows to the highs associated with various drugged and natural states.

In judging the mental status of the other person both the level of the affect on this continuum and the intensity of the feeling state are important. The appropriateness of the affect to the thought being expressed is critical to normal functioning. We usually refer to inappropriate affect as being wierd, phony, unusual, different, or silly.

ANXIETY

Anxiety is the feeling state that describes the degree of tension, restlessness, and fear that a person experiences. The interviewer can infer the level or degree of anxiety in the other person by his/her behavior, muscle tone, respiration, rate of speech, posture, and movements. The interviewer may also learn of the other persons' anxiety by statements the other person makes about him/herself. For further discussion of anxiety see pp. 60 and 81.

THINKING

Thinking is evaluated in terms of the thought content, progress of thoughts, rate, and form. In the normal individual, the flow of thoughts has a certain pace, the thoughts have an organization that can be followed and understood by the interviewer, and the thoughts are expressed in words usually associated with the thoughts. The thought flow appears logical to the observer in the normal person.

When continuous speech takes place with little or no direction, it is referred to as rambling or a flight of ideas. Words frequently used to describe abnormal progress in thinking include circumstantial, retardation, perseveration, incoherence, and blocking.

The content of thought is judged on its appropriateness to the situation. Examples of abnormal content are preoccupation of certain ideas, delusions, hypochondriacal thoughts, obsessions, phobias, and hallucinations (as illustrated by a patient who talks only about her headache the day after her husband's desertion).

SENSORIUM

Sensorium refers to the group of mental functions of the person that relate to his/her immediate intellectual integrity. In order to evaluate the person's intellectual integrity, the interviewer uses the *problem question.*

A problem question requests the person to use some aspect of his/her mental functions to answer. Examination of the sensorium usually includes evaluation of the person's mathematical ability, abstract reasoning, orientation, judgment, memory, information, and attention. Taking each of these mental functions separately, we will review ways to obtain information about the person's present functional ability.

Mathematical ability

The ability of a person to perform simple calculations mentally must be judged against the individuals educational background, current ability to concentrate on the problem, and anxiety level. Typical questions are as follows:

1. Subtract 7 from 100, then 7 from each answer you obtain.

2. If you went to the store and bought 2 cans of peas for 18 cents each and gave the grocer 50 cents, how much change would you receive?

3. How much are 7 and 6?

Abstract reasoning

There is impaired ability to think abstractly and to do abstract reasoning in persons with mental deficiency, with an acute toxic state, poisoning or head trauma. To evaluate a person's ability to reason abstractly the following questions might be used:

1. How are an apple and an orange alike?
2. How are a chair and a desk alike?
3. How are a monkey and a tree alike?

Another type of question to evaluate abstract reasoning is to ask the person to interpret the meaning of a proverb, such as:

1. What is the meaning of, "Every cloud has a silver lining?"
2. What is the meaning of, "A bird in the hand is worth two in a bush?"
3. What is the meaning of, "When the dragon goes in the water, even little fish bite its tail?"

The person's answer is judged on the basis of its relevance and degree of concreteness-abstractness.

Orientation

In both acute and chronic organic brain disorders the patient suffers from the inability to orient him/herself as to time, place, and person. A person of previously normal intelligence should know his/her age, the date, day of the week, the month, and the year. In addition, he/she should have an idea of how long it has been since breakfast or lunch and how long he/she has been in the hospital. He/she should know the city, state, and (if in the hospital) the hospital's name and should respond to and know his/her name.

Judgment

A person's judgment may be impaired as a result of organic brain dysfunction or a result of ethnic or social environment. Questions to test one's judgment are as follows:

1. If you saw $100 lying on the street corner, what would you do?
2. If you found a stamped, addressed, and sealed envelope, what would you do?
3. Ask about a situation that has occurred in the patient's own life to learn what his behavior was.
4. If a policeman stopped you for speeding, and you were sure you had not exceeded the speed limit, what would you do?

Memory

The person's recent memory may be evaluated by problem questions. Past memory may be evaluated by reviewing the consistency of his/her history. Such problem questions take place in two steps. First, the person is informed that you will give him a name, an address, and some objects that you will ask him/her for in a few minutes. For example, "My name is Dr. Arthur Brown, the address is 3635 North Beacon Street, and the objects are a tree, a table, and a desk. Now repeat them for me." You must be sure that the person has perceived the information correctly.

Next he/she is asked for other information, or other mental functions may be tested for 3 to 5 minutes. The second step is to ask: "What was the name I gave you?" (Obtain answer.) "What was the address?" (Obtain answer.) What were the objects?"

The answers are judged for accuracy, whether or not the person knew he/she was correct, and whether or not he/she made up answers to fill in for loss of memory (confabulation).

Information

A person of normal intelligence should be able to name a number of large cities, the current President and Vice President of the United States, the previous two or three Presidents of the United States, in order, and the topic of some current item of interest in the news. Failure to have this information indicates either mental deficiency, organic brain disease, or extreme social deprivation.

Attention

The person's degree of alertness and ability to participate in the interview are dependent upon his/her mental integrity. The person's attention is judged generally as part of the interview.

Question: You have just briefly examined in the emergency room a 35-year-old truck driver who received a laceration of his forehead in an automobile accident. His behavior is unusual (his speech is careless, sentences are not clear, and answers to questions are not pertinent). You want to know more about his mental abilities to confirm whether a neurosurgical or psychiatric consultation is necessary. Design an approach to test his mental ability.

Answer: Compare your answer with ours:
A. Level of attention
B. Orientation
C. Mathematical ability
D. Abstract reasoning
This evaluation should give you adequate information from which to proceed with the appropriate consultation.

Question: You have been called to a nursing home to examine an elderly physician, who is a patient, because of periods of confusion. For example, he walked into the nurse's office looking for the men's room. How would you evaluate his mental abilities?

Answer: An appropriate method would be to check the following:
A. Abstract reasoning
B. Mathematical ability
C. Orientation
D. General information
E. Memory

BEHAVIOR

When determining mental status, behavior is considered as overt gross behavior. For example, has the patient been arrested frequently, performed uncalled for or unusual acts, responded differently from others to the same employers, or has his behavior been dominated by aggressiveness, hostility, passiveness, dependency, alcohol, or drugs?

ASKING ABOUT SUICIDE

Question: You have just obtained from a person a history that leads you to believe that he/she might be seriously depressed and considering suicide. Which of the following would you use to inquire about the patient's potential for suicide?

A. Have you considered taking your life?

B. How upset are you?

C. Are you so unhappy that you feel life is not worth living?

D. What do you see in the future?

E. Are you afraid that you might hurt yourself?

F. Do thoughts about suicide bother you?

Answer: An interviewer often fears that he/she will plant the idea of suicide in the person's head. This feeling is not necessarily founded in fact. A is blunt and may not obtain a reliable reply from the person. Nevertheless it is better to ask awkwardly about suicide than not to ask at all. B and D are too open-ended to be sure that they will lead to the desired information. C, E, and F are about as specific as one can be in probing this topic with a first question.

Question: If the person answers questions C, E, and F above with "no," how do you interpret his reply?

Answer: To understand the meaning of this reply you must utilize all the nonverbal clues available to you—facial expression, position, respiration rate, pulse rate (if evident in the neck), blinking, eye movement, sweat, or bodily movement.

Question: If the person answers C, E, and F above with a "yes," how would you proceed?

Answer: Compare your response with ours:
Have you thought about suicide?
After having a "yes" to your previous question, you are invited by the person to discuss the topic further. Direct questioning about suicide is felt to be unobjectionable once it is established that the person is quite depressed. For example, he/she may express thoughts that he/she is no good, that life is not worth living, that there is no way out of the situation, or that his/her illness is hopeless.

Question: How do you interpret a "yes" and a "no" to your question, "Have you thought about suicide?"

Answer: If the person answers "yes," increased understanding will result from knowing what his/her thoughts have been. From the degree of the patient's organization, from his/her planning, and from the reasons for suicide, one may judge the degree of suicidal risk. If the person answers "no," there is still great uncertainty about suicide. Most people have thought about suicide at some time in their life. So a "no" to this question, after receiving a "yes" to the previous question, should leave the interviewer uneasy. One might challenge the "no" and judge the person's verbal and nonverbal replies, but there is no clear route to follow.

Additional practice exercises dealing with suicide are available.* Four self-administered clinical exercises are published using the invisible ink process for sequential disclosure of information as it is requested by the student. The series is designed to allow the user to assess his/her clinical abilities through simulated problems.

---

*Froelich, R. E.: Interaction strategy problems, Bowie, Maryland, 1975, Charles Press Publishers, Inc.

CHAPTER 8

NONVERBAL COMMUNICATION

ADJUVANT DATA

Adjuvant data are supporting information available to the interviewer about the patient. Examples are observations of the patient's posture, behavior, style of dress, and voice quality and modulation and the interviewer's own reactions to the patient. These observations are usually noted both consciously and unconsciously but are rarely recorded in the medical history.

In medicine, "adjuvant" refers to a substance added to a drug to aid the operation of the principal ingredient. In the interview, adjuvant data are aids to the medical history. They generally cannot stand alone and be meaningful. However, when coupled with the medical history they enhance the interviewer's understanding of the patient and either confirm or modify the diagnosis. The ability to utilize accurate adjuvant data distinguishes the skilled clinician from the mediocre one.

Posture

When presenting a patient, the student is often asked by a professor, "Did the patient appear to be sick?" The answer to this question is based on observations of the patient's posture and body movements that signal to others, "I am sick." Examples are facial expressions, alertness or dullness of the eyes, position of the head, frequency and speed of movements, and overall body position such as being doubled over or guarding and protecting a part of the body. Body posture can also serve as adjuvant data to corroborate emotional states such as depression, anxiety, dependency, suspiciousness, and elation.

Voice

The patient's voice quality suggests his/her usual method and style of relating to others. From the soft, childish tone to the loud, combative pitch are many gradations of passivity and aggression. The interviewer should differentiate between the monotone of the depressed patient and the rapid, expressive manner of the manic patient. If you begin to listen to what the tone of voice, the inflection, the pacing, and the breathing style are saying, you may perceive other important aspects about the patient.

Dress

By the manner of dress, a patient communicates his/her self-image and how he/she wishes others would relate to him/her. One useful frame of reference for understanding your observations about a patient's dress is noting its utility, its symbolism, and its appeal.* The utility of dress is its appropriateness to the task or function it is intended to serve—for example, the dressing gown for the physical examination, the tennis shorts for the game of tennis, and the space suit for the astronaut. The symbolism of dress is usually emblematic of a particular cultural-social grouping. Examples of symbolism in dress are the white coat of the medical student, the business suit for the executive, and the uniform of the doorman. The appeal of dress refers to the effect the dress has upon others and on the wearer. Examples of appeal are the feeling of sterility conveyed by hospital whites, the suggestiveness of the Playboy Bunny costume, and the rejection of the dirty, torn, hippie attire.

Question: What does it mean when a lawyer who entered the hospital 3 days ago following a myocardial infarction is seen wearing:
A. A hospital gown and robe
B. Plain pajamas and robe
C. Colorful pajamas and a decorative robe

Answer: A. He is wearing this dress for its utility. This may indicate that he doesn't care to or doesn't feel like doing anything more about clothing. The hospital gown does not signal the wearer's social position, which he has given up for the moment in becoming a patient. Consider the style of dress you would expect a colonel to wear in a military hospital. Could he give up his rank and social position and wear the same gown as an enlisted man?
B. He is wearing clothing as a symbol of his social group. In our experience, this is the usual attire for a middle- to upper-class lawyer.
C. He is wearing clothing for their appeal and pleasing quality to himself and others, as well as a symbol of the more affluent social group. It may be an attempt to be more attractive and pleasing to staff and visitors. It might even be an attempt to deny illness.

Interviewer's feelings

An interviewer can learn to use his/her own reactions as an assessment of the nature of the person who is the patient. Patients evoke feelings within interviewers, feelings of discomfort, anger, pleasure, helplessness, uneasiness, tension, boredom, or embarrassment. Physiologic reactions may include a flush, increased heart rate, change in respiration, headache, sexual arousal, tightening of the jaws, or change in peristalsis. By noting the type of patient that generates a specific reaction in yourself, you can begin to learn which reactions are diagnostic and which are nondifferential.

As with other diagnostic nosology, recognition of types of patients who

---

*Laver, J.: Modesty in dress, Boston, 1969, Houghton Mifflin Co.

consistently evoke a specific feeling is useful in planning the management of your patient and his/her illness. For example, a patient who creates anger may be the type of patient who will not carry through with a treatment program of self-medication. The patient who elicits amiable feelings may be the type of patient who overdoes everything and takes more medication than is prescribed.

Being aware of reactions to a patient assists the interviewer in consciously dealing with the feelings rather than reacting with unawareness. As an illustration, when anger is generated by a patient, the interviewer could better discharge his/her feelings by discussing them with a peer or assistant than by being abrupt with the patient.

NONVERBAL COMMUNICATION

Nonverbal communication may be defined as *all channels of communication* between two humans other than the literal meaning of the words being spoken.

Question: Which of the following could be considered nonverbal communication?
  A. Voice inflection, tone, and volume
  B. Gesture and posture
  C. Touch
  D. Dress and grooming
  E. Physical distance
  F. Facial expression
  G. Skin color (pale, blushing, dehydrated, etc.)
  H. Body hygiene

Answer: All of the above communicate something about the person nonverbally. The nonverbal communications place the verbal communication into a context, give the words additional meaning, and on occasion belie the true meaning (which may be the opposite of the verbal words) of what the speaker honestly feels or thinks. One common example is when a person makes a positive statement and simultaneously is shaking his/her head "no." Which do you believe? The verbal or the nonverbal communication? Do actions really speak louder than words?

Those who study communication have several beliefs that seem to be justified:
  1. A communication has little meaning out of context. One must know the sender, the context, and the intended receiver to know the full meaning of the communication.
  2. A student in a class must listen to the same lecturer for an average of 8 hours before the student can fully understand the lecturer. The greater the differences in cultural and ethnic backgrounds, the more hours required to reach full understanding.
  3. The most significant aspect of a message is that part of the message assimilated by the receiver.

What are the implications of these beliefs upon the practices of the health professional?

Question: Applying the first belief, that the context of the message gives the message meaning, consider the statement "My stomach hurts." What does this statement mean in each of the following circumstances?

A. A seventh grade student speaking to her mother at 8:00 A.M. on a school morning on the day of a test for which preparation has been incomplete.

B. A 35-year-old executive speaking to a physician during an emergency appointment. The executive has not been in a doctor's office in 6 years and has had no prior medical complaints. She got word yesterday that her husband was suing for divorce.

C. A 73-year-old retired college professor speaking to his physician 2 weeks after having an ulcer attack.

Answer: Each of these statements might be translated as follows (other translations may be equally valid):

A. Mother, do I have to go to school today? or Will you let me stay home?

B. I need someone to show some interest in me.

C. I believe that my stomach still hurts even after taking the medication.

The second belief, about understanding a lecturer, may be more obvious yet more difficult to document. Each patient is unique in his/her use of language to describe symptoms. Some patients describe in great detail very precise awarenesses of sensations; others rarely complain of an uncomfortable sensation. Before we can understand the meaning of the patient's words, we must have some knowledge of the person and his/her ethnic and cultural background.

Question: What would it mean to a patient if you said, "Your next appointment will be at 10 A.M. on the sixth of next month."

Answer: The statement would mean different things to different people, depending on their cultural expectations.* Some patients might interpret this statement to mean that they should arrive at the office before noon on the sixth. Others would be likely to arrive at 9:45 on the sixth. Still others might interpret the statement to mean that they should come if any discomfort persists; if there is no discomfort, there is no obligation to come.

The third belief, that the most significant aspect of a message is that part of the message assimilated by the receiver, is an important element in the treatment of a patient.

Question: What would it mean to a patient if you said, "Take one of these pills when the pain becomes severe."

Answer: Possible meanings to the patient might be:
The professional wants me to suffer some.

---

*Saunders, L.: Cultural difference and medical care, New York, 1954, Russel Sage Foundation.

The pills are powerful so don't take very many of them.
Never take two pills at one time.
Don't try to relieve the pain in any other way.
The pills will relieve any kind of pain.
The pills only work on severe pains.
Don't take the pills unless you just have to.
Take only these pills, no others, for pain.
The pain is important, tend to it carefully.

The difference between what we mean to say, what we say, and how it is interpreted is often surprising. See the section on the Purpose of an Interview for an exercise in "making meaning."

IMPORTANCE OF NONVERBAL MESSAGES

There are several possible ways that reading the patient's nonverbal messages will help you in the interview.

1. You will have a more accurate understanding of what the patient means when he/she is talking.
2. Nonverbals give instantaneous information. You don't have to wait for the end of a statement to learn the speaker's meaning.
3. If your reading of the nonverbal messages tells you whether the patient is sad, mad, glad, scared, or anxious, your response to the patient can be appropriate to the patient's feelings state (affect). For example, your response to a sad person would be quite different from your response to an angry person. If you do not read nonverbals, you may not be aware of the affect of the patient.
4. The patient's instantaneous reaction to your last action or response may be available to you only through the reading of nonverbal clues. As an on-going process without the constant nonverbal feedback the interaction may enter into mutual monologues with each of you expressing yourself as though the other were not present.
5. When you give the patient such complete attention that you read his/her nonverbals, the patient is flattered, feels positively toward you, and feels that he/she has finally found someone who can understand. When such positive rapport exists, malpractice suits are extremely rare, faithful patients are the rule, enjoyment in the practice is common, and night calls to clarify misunderstanding are rare.
6. The patient is impressed when he/she is the center of your attention. Your concern, care, and interest for the patient are apparent. Who can fail to want to cooperate when this kind of attention is being given?
7. A patient appreciates your concern for him/her as a human being, a person rather than a disease, a body, a medical rarity, or a medical challenge.
8. The information that you obtain simultaneously through more than one channel of communication is more reliable than information from a single channel. The words alone of a message may mislead, just as nonverbal clues used alone may mislead. When touch, sounds, words, body language, gestures, and facial expressions are all considered together, the true meaning of a communication is rarely missed. Each clue either substantiates your impression from the previous clue or contradicts the previous clue.

FRAMEWORK FOR READING NONVERBAL MESSAGES

It is helpful to have a framework within which meaning can be given to nonverbal clues. An effective method of organizing the information is to consider whether a person is being open or closed to a new idea or thought when he/she expresses the nonverbal message. Another method is to organize the information according to the affect (feeling) of the individual when he/she expresses a certain nonverbal message.

Open versus closed

A person is open to an idea or thought when he/she has some comfort and security with the situation, does not feel too threatened or too anxious, and has the energy necessary to consider something new. A person who is too exhausted, in too much pain, too scared, too angry, or too sad will not be open to a new idea or thought. Frequently, these internal states are reflected by body postures.

Question: Determine whether the body posture in each of the following drawings suggests that the person is open or closed to a new idea or thought.

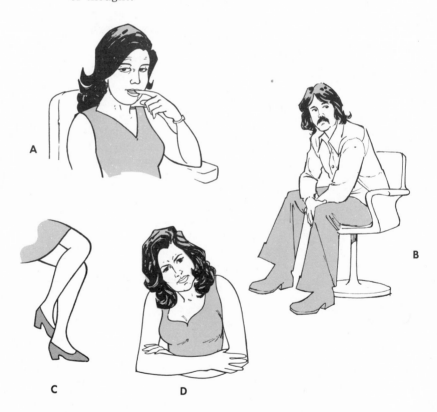

Answer: Drawings A and B are considered by most observers to be the postures that signal openness to a new idea and thought. The remaining postures are considered closed. Persons in these postures are much less frequently open to a new idea.

In the office a patient's open or closed posture may be especially important when you are ready to give the patient instructions concerning his/her treatment.

Question: If you are ready to give instructions and find that the patient is in a closed posture, what do you do?

Answer: Determine what the patient is thinking about, what is on his/her mind, and deal with the problem at hand until the patient shifts position to a more open posture. Then give your instructions. If the patient does not move to a more open posture, ask the patient if he/she is ready for the instructions about further treatment.

Question: What position do you want the patient to be in when you give instructions concerning the treatment? Should the patient be lying down, sitting up, or standing? Should the patient be above your eye level, at your eye level, or below your eye level?

Answer: Generally, you want to talk to the rational, computer part of the patient when you give him/her directions.

If the patient is lying down, he/she tends to be in a dependent, child-like ego state. If you give directions to this part of the patient, he/she may react to the directions in much the same way that a child would.

At the other extreme, if you have the patient standing over you, above you, or in a more controlling position he/she tends to be in a dominant, parent-like ego state. The patient may then react to your directions much as a parent would to directions given by a child.

Thus, directions will have greater chance of being carried out in a rational manner if they are given to the patient when he/she is seated at a height equal to yours. When the patient is at an equal height, in an upright position, he/she tends to be in the adult or computer ego state and will tend to react in a more rational manner.*

Affectual states

Your reactions to the patient will differ depending upon both the mood or affect of the patient and your own mood or affect at the time. Therefore, it is useful to have some paradigm by which moods or affects can be identified. Plutchik† has developed one useful paradigm. According to Plutchik, the primary affectual states are the unpleasurable states of sadness, anxiety, anger, and disgust; the state of comfort; and the pleasurable states of happiness, joy, and excitement.

---

*For a discussion of ego states, see James, M., and Jongeward, D.: Born to win, Reading, Mass., 1971, Addison-Wesley Pub. Co.
†Plutchik, R.: The emotions: Facts, theories, and a new model, New York, 1962, Random House Inc.

Most observers, with no training, have little difficulty reading the pleasurable affective states of happiness, joy, and excitement. Because greater difficulty more frequently occurs in reading the unpleasurable affectual states of sadness, anxiety, anger, and disgust, the interviewer may react inappropriately to the situation. For example, the interviewer's reaction to a sad person would be quite different from his/her reaction to a person who is angry.

Anxiety. Anxiety, or fear, is a common affective state. It arises from a real or imagined threat. The threat may be loss of a job, health, life, or love. The threat may be real (that is, observed by others to exist) or it may be imagined (that is, believed by the individual but unable to be observed by others). Real threats include events such as an automobile coming toward you, a hand holding a hypodermic needle coming toward you, or a barking dog lunging toward you. Imagined threats may include unconfirmed beliefs such as your boss mistrusting you, your spouse loving another person, or you having a dreaded disease.

Question: Which of the following words would the anxious person use to describe him/herself? "I am . . ."
    A. shy
    B. annoyed
    C. sad
    D. tired
    E. nervous
    F. anxious
    G. apprehensive

Answer: A, E, F, and G are words frequently used by the anxious person.

Question: How would the anxious person complete the following sentence? "I feel like . . ."
    A. hitting
    B. running
    C. shaking
    D. going away
    E. vomiting
    F. laughing
    G. hiding

Answer: B, C, E, and G are feelings frequently expressed by the anxious person.

Question: Select the drawings in each of the following pairs that best portray anxiety.

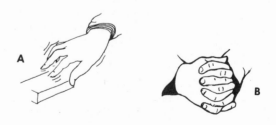

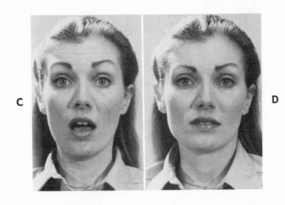

C   D

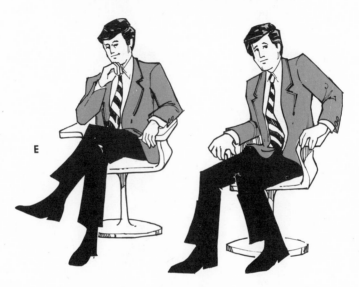

E

Answer: A, C, and F best portray anxiety. The anxious facial expression
may include a raised forehead, raised eyebrows, eyelids open
wide to see from where the danger is coming, dilated pupils,
a round, open mouth, trembling lips, and a licking of the lips.
In addition, the face may be white with cold sweat. The anxious
person's bodily expressions may include a fixed head, as though
he/she were pulling away, gestures of guarding him/herself,
trembling, a posture of being ready for flight, and trivial hand
occupation.

Question: What is the respiration like in the anxious person? Describe the
rate, depth of respiration, and (going back to physiology), the
efficiency of this type of breathing.

Answer: The anxious person breathes more rapidly than normal. The
depth of respiration is very shallow. When the rapid rate is
combined with the shallow excursion, little air is moved and
very little oxygen is exchanged in the alveoli. Thus, the efficiency
is decreased, and a mild anoxia exists. Some authorities believe

that if the amount of oxygen (oxygen tension) in the blood is increased in a person who is anxious, the person will feel less anxious and more comfortable.

Question: According to the last answer, what would you do to enable an anxious person to feel less anxious and more comfortable?

Answer: You would encourage the person to breathe more slowly and with deeper respirations. One technique is to have the person count to four during each of the following: inspiration, holding breath in, expiration, and holding breath out. The person should repeat the cycle until he/she is more comfortable.

Question: Which of the following drawings portrays the gait of an anxious person?

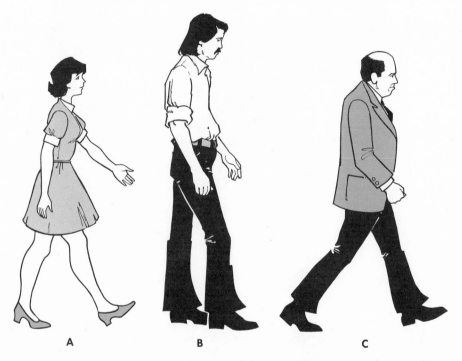

A   B   C

Answer: A depicts the gait of the anxious person. It is careful and cautious, with head erect, eyes searching for danger, and weight centered between the feet. The body is erect, and the stride is usually lengthened. The walk of the anxious person shows the energy that is in check but available.

Anger. Anger is the normal response to frustration. When progress toward a goal is impeded, a person is frustrated in moving toward the goal, he/she does not like it, and the resulting physiologic changes and behavior are described as aggression or anger. Anger resulting from stimuli that is nonobstructive (that does not interfere in reaching of goals) is considered neurotic.

Question: Which of the following drawings portray the angry person?

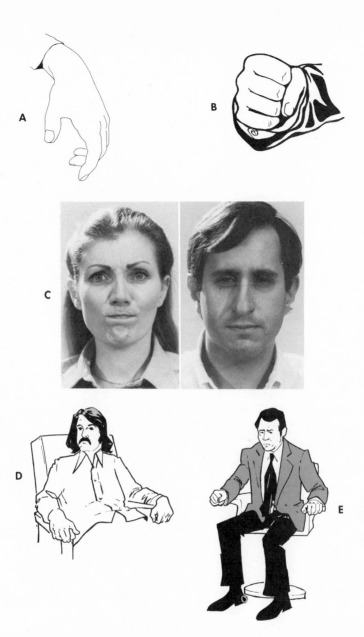

Answer: Drawings B, C, and E are examples of nonverbal expressions of anger. Note that the angry face has a frowning forehead, knit eyebrows, the lids are narrowed, and the eyes are looking straight at the barricade that impedes the progress. The mouth may be open in an elliptical, tense grin, with teeth clenched, and the lips are compressed and retracted. The neck veins are prominent (distended), the face is red, the masseter muscles are tight, and the nostrils are widened. The head is forward with the chin protruding.

Question: Which of the following words would the angry person use to describe him/herself? "I am . . ."
A. fearful
B. annoyed
C. dejected
D. in a rage
E. disinterested
F. mad
G. bad
H. irritated
I. angry

Answer: B, D, E, F, G, H, and I are words frequently used by the person who is angry.

Question: How would the angry person complete the following sentence? "I feel like . . ."
A. hiding
B. giving up
C. hitting
D. shouting
E. crying
F. slamming the door
G. killing
H. running

Answer: C, D, F, and G are feelings frequently expressed by the angry person.

Question: How would you describe the gait of an angry person?

Answer: The gait of the angry person may be portrayed by the following drawing.

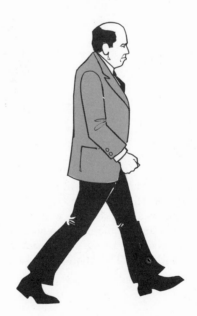

In the gait of the angry person the weight is forward, the head is forward and up so that the eyes are looking straight ahead, the muscles are set, the hands are in the form of a fist, and the arms are rigid. This person is ready to fight with the obstacle in his/her way.

Question: Describe the respiration and speech of the angry person.

Answer: The respiration is forceful with speech occuring in the middle of the expiration. The speech comes in staccato bursts or outbursts, is forceful, loud, and precise.

Grief and sorrow. Grief and sorrow are the feelings that are the normal response to loss. The loss may be that of a loved one, friend, object, part of oneself (such as a finger), pet, or position. The loss of respect, freedom, or faith may also be considered significant losses. The physiologic reaction to loss is described by the words grief, sorrow, and sadness.

Question: Which of the following words would a person use to describe him/herself when grieving or sorrowful? "I am . . ."
A. dejected
B. irritated
C. anxious
D. pensive
E. depressed
F. tired
G. gloomy
H. sad

Answer: A, D, E, G, and H are the words used by the person who is experiencing grief or sorrow.

Question: How would such a person complete the following sentence? "I am . . ."
A. giving up
B. running away
C. hitting
D. crying
E. falling apart
F. going away
G. empty
H. dying

Answer: A, D, F, G, and H are feelings frequently expressed by the person who has experienced a loss. Remember that running away is an expression of the anxious person. The sad person does not have the energy available that the anxious or angry person has.

Question: How might you help a person who has just suffered a loss to cope with the loss more effectively?

Answer: Since this person does not have much energy available, you should do anything that you can to help the person get in touch with his/her energy. First, allow the person to grieve, to cry, and to be sad, but then help the person to return to activities that are normal for him/her.

Just remember that everything we now have (friends, possessions, pets, health, mental and physical abilities) we must give up sooner or later. Many have already been given up (for example, diapers, being a child, being carried, high school, etc.). Each was a loss at the time it was given up. We survived, we coped, and we can deal with future losses.

Question: Which of the following drawings portray the person who is grieving? Select the drawings that best portrays a sad person.

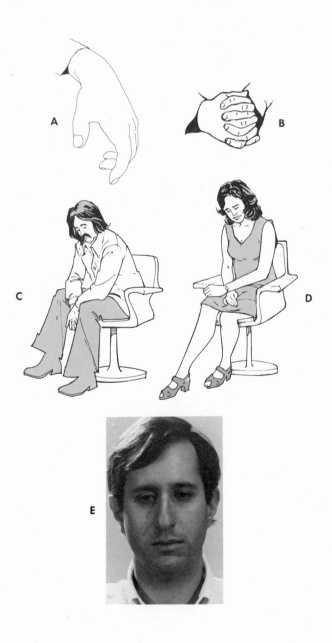

Answer: A, C, D, and E depict expressions of sorrow. The sad, grieving person has the forehead flat, eyes half closed, and downcast; the eyes may be red with tears, the mouth is in the form of an inverted cresent; the face is pale and lengthened, and the muscles are flaccid. It is as though there were no nerve impulses to the muscles of the face and they were being pulled by gravity.

Question: Describe the speech and respiration of the grieving person.

Answer: The respirations are slow, sighing, and shallow. The speech is soft, slow, and weeping, and occurs at the end of expiration. Air is exhaled in a sigh before the person speaks (toward the end of the expiration).

Question: Describe the posture and gait of the grieving person.

Answer: The posture of the sad, grieving person may be described as "the body hanging by the ligaments." It is as though there were no muscle tone or muscular help in holding the body erect. The head is hanging. The limbs are limp, there are few gestures except for some hand-wringing. The gait is slouched, weight is back on the feet, and steps tend to be short and slow. Abdominal muscles sag and the abdomen is protuberant. Arms are relaxed. It is as though the person were saying to the world, "Come hit me, for I must be bad and deserve to be punished. I am defenseless and will (can) *not* put up a fight." Another reading of this posture may be, "I am helpless, come take care of me." The following drawing depicts the gait of the sad person.

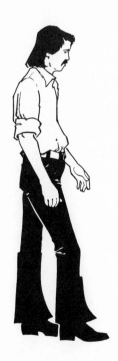

Disgust. Disgust is the physiologic response to a noxious situation or stimulus. The situation or stimulus is one with which the person can*not* be comfortable.

Question: Which of the following words would the disgusted person use to describe him/herself? "I am . . ."
- A. bored
- B. nauseated
- C. annoyed
- D. dejected
- E. tired
- F. loathing
- G. disinterested

Answer: A, B, E, and F are words frequently used by the disgusted person.

Question: How would a disgusted person complete the following sentence? "I feel like . . ."
- A. vomiting
- B. crying
- C. hiding
- D. bashing in a wall
- E. turning away
- F. running

Answer: A, C, and E are feelings expressed by the disgusted person.

Question: Which of the following drawings portray the disgusted person?

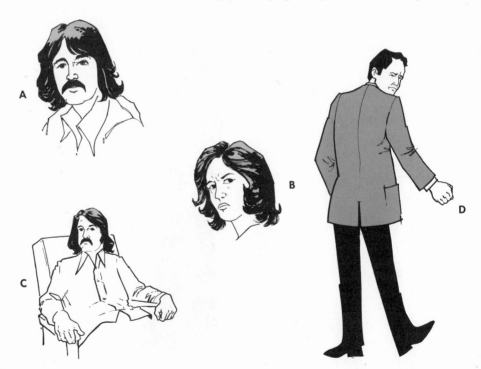

Answer: B and D represent the nonverbal expressions of disgust. The face of the disgusted person has some frowning of the forehead; the eyes squint occasionally and turn away. The mouth may show a sneer or the early signs of imminent vomiting. The head is generally turned away from the object or person associated with the disgust. The posture of the disgusted person is primarily that of turning or pushing away, with a hand moving to the abdomen or mouth as if to catch an uncomfortable part of the body.

Question: Describe the speech and respiration of the disgusted person.

Answer: The speech is snorting or sneering. The respiration is halting; there is a tendency to hesitation.

Question: When might you expect to observe a reaction of disgust?

Answer: Obviously, the reaction will occur following the presentation of something to the patient. It might be an examining instrument, a form, a treatment plan, or a recommendation for care. In these situations it may be very important to be alert to such a reaction by a patient.

Question: You just presented the treatment plan to a patient and observed a reaction that you interpret to be one of disgust. How might you proceed?

Answer: There are several ways to proceed. One way might be to comment on the patient's reaction. When you make this type of confrontation, it is best to use a congruent statement, one in which you take full responsibility for your observation of disgust, and one in which you allow the patient to deal with this reaction. You should not be critical of the reaction; the patient has every right to dislike your plan. The following responses fill these requirements:

I detect some discomfort on your part to this treatment plan.
I sense that you are not pleased with this treatment plan.

CHAPTER 9

THE COOPERATIVE PATIENT

One of the essentials that leads to having a satisfied patient is having the patient's cooperation during the course of care. The cooperative patient is one who follows directions, participates in the evaluation, takes medications that are prescribed in the manner prescribed, comes for appointments, takes appropriate care of his/herself, and so on. This type of patient cooperates with the health professional in his/her health care or management.

Some of the factors that lead to professional-patient cooperation are mutual trust, the patient's feeling that the professional cares, the patient's belief in the professional (that the professional is honest, good, competent, and concerned), mutual respect, a mutual feeling of being able to communicate and be understood, and both persons being in a "you count" position.

This chapter focuses on trust.

TRUST

What is the source of trust in one individual toward another? Why do some people trust when others in the same situation do not trust? Is a sense of personal security within the individual important to the establishment of trust?

Question: When one individual does not trust another, there are many indicators that trust does not exist. What are some of the indicators?

Answer: Hesitant speech
Guarded postures
Anxiety
Strong need to please
Inability to say no
Testing behavior to see if the other person can be trusted
Broken appointments
False airs, phoniness
A feeling of uneasiness in the presence of the other person

Once you are aware of another person's lack of trust in you, how do you go about understanding it? To understand lack of trust perhaps it is necessary to first understand trust.

Trust develops from very personal experiences that are unique for each individual. Once trust in a specific relationship develops, it can then be generalized to other individuals and to institutions.

Trust may be viewed as developing from a series of behavior predictions by one individual about another individual that are in harmony with what the other individual says he/she will do or be and then actually does or is. This predictive accuracy must be consistent over a number of experiences for an individual to develop trust in the second individual.

In the professional office the development, or lack, of trust usually depends on the actuality of what the professional says will or will not happen. If you say, "This will not hurt," whether it does or does not hurt makes a difference in the development of the patient's trust. If you say, "I will see you next Tuesday at 11:00," whether you see that patient at 11:00 or 11:20 makes a difference. Each of these situations leads to the ability of the patient to accurately predict your behavior and learn that what you say can (or cannot) be trusted.

How can a patient trust a professional who says, "This won't hurt" and then it does? Or the professional who says, "I will see you at 11:00" and then doesn't see the patient until 11:25? What should the patient do when the professional says, "Take these tablets at noon each day for 10 days." Should the patient take them at 1:00 p.m. and for 13 days? How can the patient trust what the professional says when what he/she tells the patient is not true as the patient experiences it?

Once a person can trust one other person (one health professional), then that person is more likely to transfer or generalize this trust to other persons (other health professionals) and will continue to trust until he/she finds a professional that he/she cannot trust. For most of us this development of trust, or lack of it, started before we were able to remember specific events. It started with our relationship with our parenting persons in our first year of life and continues to be tested and revised every day.

From trusting specific family members, friends, and associates, we develop a generalized level of trust in others, such as the bus driver, the airline pilot, the other driver on the street, the banker, and the government. As the list expands, we realize that our trust in many of these individuals is blind in the sense that we will never know these people as individuals or have any personal experience with them; but we will nevertheless trust them based upon a general feeling of trust for others. We trust them, however, because we have a generalized feeling of trust in others.

In some individuals, a lack of trust in others leads them to alter their life in order to avoid being placed in situations where they are forced to be dependent on the untrusted others. Some persons' refusal to fly is based upon this lack of trust in mechanics, pilots, ground controllers, electronics, machines, and so on. For a moment, consider what life would be like if you were unable to trust those around you—how you would always have to be in control of everything, leaving nothing to others, never being dependent, always being alert, never sleeping for fear that someone might harm you. Can you get a feeling of the magnitude of the burden carried by a person who has trouble trusting others?

Do not take a patient's difficulty in trusting you lightly. It is a serious problem for the patient and for you. Respect the magnitude of this problem.

Be aware that you must do what you say you will do, and that you must make accurate statements about what you expect the patient to feel or not feel as you work on him/her. Keep your appointments at the time you say; if you are delayed, get a message to the patient that you expect to see him/her in a certain number of minutes and ask whether he/she prefers to wait or be rescheduled. Your failure to carry out the contract of seeing the patient at the appointed time cancels the contract, and a new contract needs to be negotiated. Once you fail to keep the appointed time, the patient is free to leave and seek another appointment time. The patient may, out of courtesy to you, wait until you are ready to see him/her. The opposite holds true also; out of courtesy to the patient you may wait when he/she is delayed.

Trust between two persons is affected by the observations of the individuals involved. Because "believing is seeing," the person who generally trusts others will "see" that he/she can trust what you do and say. Likewise, when a person generally distrusts others, he/she will "see" distrust in what you do and say. You may have to confront such a person with the fact that although he/she did not trust you about a certain matter, in fact you did what you said you would do. Thus, it may take a very active, aggressive assault on the distrust to establish a trusting relationship.

Examples of trust

Perhaps one of the first signs of lack of trust is the failure of a patient to carry out his/her part of the treatment. For example, a patient obviously has not taken proper care of him/herself after being instructed during a previous visit.

Question: A patient has not properly cared for a cast after having been instructed in its care. What would you say to the patient to correct this situation.

Answer: You need to first establish a common understanding. The patient does not know that you think he has not followed your directions. You do not know when or how the patient failed in the care of his cast. What you do know is that the desired result has not occurred. Thus a supportive confrontation or sharing of information and beliefs is needed to establish what exactly has taken place since you last saw the patient.

Question: Which of the following would you say to the patient:
A. How have you been caring for your cast since I last saw you?
B. Something is not going as it should; your cast seems to be mashed as if you were not taking care of it. How have you cared for it?
C. How are you caring for your cast now?
D. It looks like you have been having trouble caring for your cast.
E. It looks as though you have been having trouble caring for your cast. Does that agree with what you feel?
F. Gee! This cast is torn up. Can't you care for it as I told you? There is no point in me doing any more for you until you take care of your cast.

Answer: A, B, and E support the patient and open the topic for the patient to tell you what he/she has experienced. All except for A let the patient know what you are thinking and give the patient some idea of why you are asking the questions and seeking the information.

C and D ask for very specific information, implying that you already know exactly what is the trouble.

F will drive the patient away unless you have a very secure, trusting relationship with him/her.

Question: A patient presents a very guarded posture while you are interviewing him. Which of the following would you choose to say?

A. Now, just relax.
B. There is nothing to be afraid of.
C. You seem to have become tense. Are you aware of that?
D. You seem to be uncomfortable. Am I reading you correctly?
E. You seem to be uncomfortable. Is there something we can do to make you more comfortable?
F. What are your thinking that you are becoming tense and defensive or scared?

Answer: C, D, and E tell the patient what you have noticed and ask for verification of what is going on inside.

C focuses upon the patient's awareness of internal feelings.

D does much the same thing as C but seeks to determine whether there is agreement between you concerning what the patient is feeling.

E focuses on treating the situation and by-passes any idea that your observations may be a misunderstanding of the patient's feelings.

A and B are examples of the magic of words. Say it and it will be so. The words heal. If you see your role as that of a witch doctor, select and use these responses. In practice you cannot change how another human being feels by just commanding or telling this person how he/she should feel.

F is the ideal response with a psychologically sophisticated patient. This response strikes at the heart of the problem and will lead to a correction of the tension if the patient is able to understand and control thoughts and resultant feelings. Do not use this response with a patient who has not had psychologic training in either growth experiences, personal therapy, or sensitivity-encounter group experiences.

This last response *(F)* alludes to the process of tension and the resultant defensiveness as we understand it. While the interview is going on, the patient is thinking something. When the patient changes in his/her degree of comfort or relaxation, most likely (if the interviewer has not done anything specific) the patient has had a frightening thought. Focusing on this thought will bring out all of the old fears of the patient that are associated with the thought. Focusing the patient's thoughts upon something else will change the patient's feelings and thus the patient's degree of comfort.

CHAPTER 10

FAMILY INTERVIEWING

OPENING—PURPOSE AND CONTRACT

The purpose of a family or group interview is (1) to learn how each member considers, or feels about, an issue; (2) to learn how each member relates to each other member; and (3) to obtain a common understanding within the group or family. Some of the circumstances requiring the health professional to see a family as a group are decisions regarding surgery, special treatments for cancer, the prognosis for recovery after an accident, family plans after a member has had a stroke, consideration for a nursing home placement, and marital counseling regarding sex, family planning, or divorce.

When dealing with a sick person whose illness is affected by his/her social and emotional environment, a family interview may be most helpful in understanding the stresses to which the patient is reacting. Many times the illness is the manifest issue but the problem that must be dealt with is the communication patterns that have developed within the family. The scapegoat of a family is an easily understood illustration that our society recognizes and even names. The scapegoat has many more illnesses than do his/her peers in the family.

Question: What would be wrong with opening your first session with a family or group in each of the following ways?
A. Silence while awaiting a member of the group to speak.
B. What is the situation that brings you here?
C. It is good to see you. What is on your mind?

Answer: A. Silence in the opening of a group session leads to anxiety and hostility within the group. There is no reason here to generate anxiety or hostility at the beginning of the session. The hostility is usually directed toward the leader and may indeed create a barrier to further useful communication.
B and C. If the health professional were caught off guard or surprised by a family or group, opening with *B* or *C* might be appropriate. However, in most circumstances one member of the group or the family in consultation with the health professional has arranged for the meeting, or the health

professional has arranged it directly. The health professional is the leader of the group and has the responsibility for its direction. He/she has the responsibility to define why the group has been asked to assemble and the purpose of the meeting. An alternative is to have each person state what he/she believes to be the reason for the meeting. This latter approach places hidden agendas out in the open.

Question: Make up an opening for a family group session called together to help a family make realistic plans for the 68-year-old father who has had a stroke. Since the patient's stroke, you have had brief casual contacts with all of the family members.

Answer: Compare your opening statement with the following:
I have asked that we meet together to consider your father's (use the patient's name, never "the patient's") stroke and the best way to manage his care when he leaves the hospital. Since I have talked with all of you at one time or another, I wonder what possible plans you have considered.

This opening has several aspects:
1. The responsibility for the meeting is clearly stated by the health professional. (This avoids any possible friction between family members that might arise from feelings that one of them called the meeting to gain a special position of power or control over who takes care of father.)
2. The purpose of the meeting is clearly stated.
3. The statement that you have talked with each member of the family does not single out one for a special position of power.
4. Finding the solution to the problem is shared with them by asking, "What possible plans have you considered?"

In summary, with this opening the interviewer accepts responsibility, takes charge of the meeting, treats the members as equals, and treats them on an adult level, expecting them as a group to solve the problem with the health professional's assistance.

PATIENT INCLUSION

Question: Should father be present during this joint interview?

Answer: There is no single answer if his physical condition does not prevent his being present. To have father present at the sessions shows him respect, directly reinforces how much concern there is for him, and makes him a part of the decision-making group. Father may be upset by being dependent. If so, a session with the family is one way to help him see that the family feels he is worth the time and trouble and that they plan to help him grow more independent as he recovers from his stroke. Acceptance of one's dependency needs, if first confronted with illness at 68 years of age, is not easy and will take some adjustment by father. Seeing the family as a group will avoid misinterpretations and misunderstandings of what the health professional may say. In seeing father or any member of the family alone, what the health professional said may be reported incorrectly, and there is no one to correct the error. In a group session misinterpretations are corrected by other family members who were present.

OPENNESS

If one of the goals in the family management is to obtain more openness, more honesty, and greater freedom in the communication among family members, having father present and included in the discussion will set the stage for open communication about the problem at hand.

If expression of feelings is encouraged during the session, family members may learn that such expression has more positive than negative results. If brother John's wife is upset by her father-in-law's presence and could never share directly in his care, this should be known and accepted by the group. Once the feeling is in the open, John's wife may then be able to contribute to his care in ways that do not involve personal contact.

If the feeling is not discussed, some family members may feel put upon, jealous, used, or angry toward John's wife. With discussion, the jealous, angry feelings may still be present, but at least an attempt is made to find some constructive way that John's wife can contribute to father's care.

A reason for not having father present during the session would be any impairment preventing him from following and understanding what is said. A hearing defect, an associative defect from brain damage, or mental confusion from the stroke would all suggest that being present may be more upsetting than useful.

If you are aware that one of the family members is extremely hostile toward father, you may decide to deal with the hostility before father is present. On the other hand, it might be constructive to confront the family openly with the hostility. This would demonstrate that hostility is not extremely frightening, that it can be dealt with, and that hostility can be seen as a form of caring about the other person.

COMMUNICATION PATTERNS

Question: In addition to the factual data gathered from what is said, what else do you look for in a joint interview?

Answer: You look for the types of communication patterns used by the various members of the family.*

Question: The following communication styles may emerge during the group session. Compliant statements are: "If that is what you want to do, it is okay with me." "Whatever you say is fine." "I'll go along with whatever the group decides." Describe this person's position in the group. Is he/she making a positive contribution or taking any responsibility for the group's decision?

Answer: He/she is avoiding any responsibility for the group decision. He/she is being passive and compliant and tends to be a neutral rather than a constructive force within the group.

Question: Accusative statements are: "Why do you always come up with that kind of a solution?" "You always want things your way." "You never agree with whatever is said." "Why do you always

---

*Satir, V.: People making, Palo Alto, Ca., 1972, Behavior Books, Inc.

look at the negative side?" What effect will statements of this type have in a group?

Answer: Accusative statements in a group are never constructive. They are disruptive of the group process and tend to prevent the successful accomplishment of the task. They tend to put the others on the defensive. This person is finding fault with what is being done and by this approach offers no constructive comments to the task at hand.

Question: Blaming statements are: "You always take his side." "If it weren't for your failure to help father, he wouldn't be where he is today." "You should make up your mind what you want to do." "If you hadn't insisted upon your way last week, things would be different." What does a person accomplish with these statements?

Answer: Such statements tend to express hostility and divide the group. They challenge the person to whom they are directed and place that person on the defensive. Such statements do not lead to a constructive solution of the task at hand.

Question: The intellectualizer usually makes statements such as: "In one study I read, 40 percent of the stroke patients did better by . . ." "According to Dr. King, father should have . . ." "In *Time Magazine* last week, a survey showed . . ." What do statements like these tend to do to the communication process in a group?

Answer: These statements take the conversation away from the specific situation and focus upon more abstract data, situations, and treatment. They may challenge the health professional. The person making the statements can do so and not accept any responsibility for the statement. He/she can always cite the authors of the statements and hold them responsible.

Question: Irrelevant statements are: "The weather looks threatening." "What time do you need to be at the game?" "I like that tie." "Mary, how long have you had that dress?" What is the effect of such statements?

Answer: They disrupt concentration on the topic being discussed. They are especially disruptive to the person to whom they are addressed. They show a lack of interest in the topic being discussed by the group. They also indicate that the speaker is either incapable of dealing with the topic or is trying to avoid the topic. Jokes are usually irrelevant, although they frequently break tension and allow the group to relax and go on. In this use, irrelevant statements are constructive.

Question: A healthy or congruent communication style has a unique form. It consists of a statement about how the speaker feels or what he/she thinks about the topic and then asks for others to state their position. For example: "I believe that father should stay with Mary when he leaves the hospital. What do the rest of you think?" "I would like mother to express what she feels should be done.

What do the rest of you feel?" "I do not believe that father would be happy living with John. What do you think?" What is the effect of these statements?

Answer: The result of such statements is that once each has made his/her position known, the group can work from this knowledge toward a reasonable solution. Only when the members are using a healthy or congruent communication style can the group complete the task at hand. One blamer or accusative person can prevent the group from reaching a decision.

While these behaviors are discussed relative to family or group interviewing, they are also relevant to committee meetings and other interactions of task-oriented groups.

OTHER OBSERVATIONS

Question: What other factors should be considered during a group session?

Answer: Who takes control? Who may be in control even without speaking? Where does each member sit? Whom does each one sit next to? Does any member of the group feel left out? Has everyone had an opportunity to speak or be called on? Has concern and interest been shown for each person's thoughts and feelings? If not, before you allow the session to end you should invite the silent members of the group to comment.

Question: How would you phrase the statement to call on the silent members, John and Sue, for a comment?

Answer: Did your statement show them your concern? Did it show interest in them? Did your statement address them by name? Compare your response with ours:
John, you haven't said anything. I would like to know how you see (feel about) the group's decision.
I would like to know what Sue thinks about our discussion.
Sue, since you haven't said anything, I don't know where you stand on this topic. I would like to know.

These suggested responses confront the member of the group with his/her silence, show your interest and concern, and take the responsibility for inviting him/her to speak. You need to know where each person stands and whether or not he/she will support the group's decision.

PART THREE

INFLUENCES UPON THE INTERVIEW

CHAPTER 11

INITIAL CONTACTS WITH OTHERS

The patient has decided to contact the office for medical care. Consider for a moment the patient's state of mind.

Question: How would you describe the patient's state of mind? (How do you feel when you are about to embark upon a new experience in a new territory?)

Answer: The most universal reaction to a new situation or new people at a time when you are asking for help, feeling a little helpless, and needing to depend upon someone else whom you don't yet know is anxiety. The degree of anxiety depends upon a number of variables: How many different experiences with new people have you encountered before? (Did you grow up in a community where you knew everyone and rarely met a stranger?) How secure are you within yourself? Are you really okay? Can you really handle any situation? What thoughts do you have about the new situation that might scare you?

Some patients will feel trapped and intruded on because they have to break their routine and go to an office. They don't like the intrusion into their life. They are annoyed and frustrated because the appointment prevents them from continuing toward their planned goal. They may be angered. They don't like being sick, having pain, or not being perfect. So the receptionist may be confronted with anger, unexplained aggression, irritability, or a contrary patient.

Still other patients will view their need for care as a loss of their integrity, a loss of their wholeness, a loss of their power and possibly a loss of their youth. These patients will react with some degree of grief and sadness. Their spirits will be down, and there may be some slowing of their normal physiologic functioning. Extreme slowing of physiologic functioning leads to coating of the tongue, constipation, decreased salivation, dryness of the mouth, slowed movements such as gait, gestures, speech. This extreme slowing will not occur from just the need for an appointment, but if the appointment is part of other losses, such as from a death, business loss, divorce, or the like, the changes in the general physiology may lead to changes easily recognized. Examples of these changes can be found in state mental hospitals in people who have had long periods of altered physiologic responses.

Question: With the patient in a state of mind somewhere within the range of feelings just reviewed, what is the job of the receptionist when the phone rings?

Answer: The receptionist's job is to establish communication with the prospective patient in such a way that the appointment will be made and kept.

Question: Assume that the patient is experiencing some anxiety and has some of the other feelings. What does the prospective patient want to hear on the telephone?

Answer: The patient wants the telephone voice on the other end to be concerned, accepting, warm, and friendly rather than cold, distant, and businesslike.

Question: Select the way(s) listed below that you believe an office telephone should be answered:
A. 3454673.
B. Hello.
C. Doctor's office.
D. Dr. Howard West's office, Kathy speaking.
E. Dr. Howard West's office, Kathy Arnold speaking.
F. Dr. West's office, Ms. Arnold speaking.
G. Dr. West's.
H. Dr. West's office, may I help you?

Answer: We prefer D, E, and F.
A is cold and distant.
B doesn't inform you whether or not you have reached the correct doctor's office.
C could very easily be inferred as "Hello, stop bothering me."
G is a step in the right direction but continues to be impersonal.
H is friendly, gives information, and is acceptable.
We prefer for the receptionist to give his/her name. When the receptionist gives his/her name, the caller usually does likewise without having to be asked for it. When we give our names, we are saying that we are individuals, that we are not ashamed of our name, that we stand behind our name, and, by inference, that we stand behind what we do. Giving our name makes our conversations personal rather than impersonal. It also implies that we deal with unique individuals with names, not with abstract, depersonalized patients.

The next job of the receptionist is to obtain the caller's name and request. The receptionist needs to record the request as accurately as possible, because what the caller says contains clues as to his/her state of mind, the real purpose of the appointment (not just the stated purpose), and what concerns the caller has.

Question: How should the receptionist ask the patient for the reason for the appointment?

    A. Why do you want the appointment?

    B. What trouble do you have?

    C. What is bothering you?

    D. What may I record as your reason for the appointment?

    E. May I indicate on your record your reason for the appointment?

Answer: D and E are the preferred answers. These questions infer that the receptionist will listen to what is said in reply, is concerned with what is about to be said, and will write down what is said. They suggest that no judgment will be made regarding the legitimacy of the patient's request for an appointment.

A tends to be accusative and places the patient in a defensive position to justify the request for an appointment.

B and C are too superficial for a professional setting.

Question: Consider each of the following responses to the receptionist's question, "What may I record as your reason for the appointment?" Which patient is anxious? Which patient is angry? Which patient is sad?

    A. I (pause) I have a headache. (Said at the beginning of expiration.)

    B. I need an appointment for my headache. (Said forcefully.)

    C. My head hurts. (Said slowly at the end of expiration.)

Answer: A is anxious.

    B is angry.

    C is sad.

Note that the pause and how the voice sounded are part of the communication and need to be recorded by the receptionist. The hesitations, voice quality, respiration, and other nonverbal clues may be more important than what the patient says, in terms of how soon you see the patient, how you deal with the patient, and what treatment you recommend. If the patient is so angry that his tight muscles about his forehead are causing his headache, the usual treatment plan may have to be altered. But more important, you might not want to make jokes with the angry patient or expect the sad patient to actively pursue exercises. You know that the anxious, somewhat hysterical patient, on the other hand, will overdo your suggestions in an attempt to please you.

The receptionist should get the available information from the patient and make sure that the patient feels welcome and cared for, so that the patient will keep the appointment and be in a state of mind that is conducive to good care.

There are differing opinions concerning the correct method and style to be used by the professional in meeting a new patient and in establishing an interview relationship of trust and confidence.

Do you personally escort the patient from the waiting room?

Do you have the patient wait in the office?

Do you first see the new patient in a private office setting?

Do you shake hands or do you ignore this social convention?

Do you talk about the weather or do you get right to the problem?

There is no single answer to these questions since no single practice is accepted by all professionals.

In the next frames assume that you (a patient) have just moved to a new city.

After telephoning an office and being told to come right in and you will be seen, you enter the office. The receptionist takes your name, address, occupation, complaint, and other information. She hangs up your coat and places you in the consultation room and leaves. You wait for 50 minutes and the health professional enters.

Question: As a patient, what is your reaction to this introduction to the office?

Answer: This introduction may leave you feeling that the office has an efficient receptionist, but wondering if anyone has any interest in you.

Remember, many patients consider evidence of interest in them as a criterion of scientific competence. Every cultural group considers it insulting to be kept waiting beyond a certain period of time without some additional communication from office personnel. With alertness, the staff can determine what this time limit is for the individual community where the practice is located.

After telephoning a second office and being told to come right in and you will be seen, you enter the office. The receptionist obtains the necessary information and asks you to be seated in the waiting room. In approximately 10 minutes the receptionist checks with the health professional and tells you that he will be delayed in seeing you, and can she make you more comfortable while you wait. After another 15 minutes the health professional introduces himself to you at the waiting room door, escorts you to the consultation room, and takes your coat.

Question: As a patient, what is your reaction to this introduction to the office?

Answer: This introduction shows interest and respect on the part of the staff. You are kept informed about a delayed time schedule. You know the staff is aware of your existence and uncomfortable state.

After telephoning a third office to ask about help, you are told that you can be seen at 4:45 p.m. but if you become too uncomfortable you may come in earlier and wait until you can be worked into the schedule. You enter the office 5 minutes before your appointment time. The receptionist obtains the necessary information. She hangs up your coat and places you in a consultation room. The health professional enters at 4:47 and introduces herself.

Question: As a patient, what is your reaction to this introduction to the office?

Answer: This introduction shows concern about the value of the patient's time and understanding that the patient must weigh the degree of discomfort against waiting time in the office. You may appreciate the promptness and businesslike approach of the staff. Whether the health professional is a cold, unfeeling technician or a warm, understanding person will be shown by how he/she proceeds from here.

Each office develops a pattern of dealing with patients. Sometimes this evolves by chance and with little or no thought given to the impression it gives to the patient. The staff should be aware of the way the patient is managed, including the initial telephone contact, when the patient arrives at the office, and during the initial face-to-face meeting with the patient. First impressions are too important to be left to chance.

Discussions about these last three examples, and others you may think of, will further your understanding of how the patient reacts to the office introductions. Such discussions will improve your control of the introduction patterns developed in your office.

The relationship between the staff and the patient is not a social one; the roles of the staff and the patient are defined by cultural definitions and expectations. The relationship is defined as a professional-client one, with certain reciprocal rights and privileges denied social relationships. Some professionals feel strongly that, from the outset, the behavior of the professional should clearly indicate that the relationship is a professional one. It has a purpose that is agreed to by both the patient and the health professional and rarely is some social exchange necessary to begin the diagnostic-helping interview. If the patient is unusually anxious, apprehensive, or frightened, then an element of social amenity might not be remiss.

Question: When meeting a new patient in your office, would you shake hands?

Answer: Social handshaking occurs primarily when two men meet initially or when they have been apart for some time. Shaking hands is much less frequent among women although it is presently increasing as a feminine behavior. Shaking hands in an office is not common. After all, it is not a sociable relationship. On the other hand, you may obtain some valuable information that can be exchanged from the handshake (whether the patient's hand is limp or firm, wet or dry, steady or shaking, clumsy or agile, deformed or normal) and can transmit your reaction to the patient (concern, support, considerateness, firmness, tenderness, or distance). The rule is to *shake hands if it is the comfortable thing* for you and for the patient to do.

CHAPTER 12

OFFICE SETTINGS

OFFICE ENVIRONMENT

As the patient enters a new environment, his/her impression is based on the total sensory experience—temperature, colors, texture, sounds, location, dress, and artifacts. Some offices strive for the formal setting, whereas others strive for the informal. Either an efficient long-life, strong, durable, hard surfaced rug or a soft, fluffy, well padded inviting rug may be placed on the waiting room floor. The magazines may be *Playboy, Better Homes and Gardens, Popular Mechanics, Field and Stream, Children's Highlights,* or *National Geographic* depending on your clientele. An inappropriate magazine for the social or ethnic class may attract or repel patients as much as your technical skills.

Do you want to have games in the waiting room? Should you always have a half-finished puzzle on the table? What do you want patients to do while waiting for you? Do you want to distract their thoughts? Do you want to have them worry about what will happen to them today? The waiting room may be a significant factor concerning how the patient will first respond to you.

Question: What do you want to say with your waiting room?
   A. This is a place of business, we are all business.
   B. We are friendly and are concerned with your comfort.
   C. You are welcome. Come and be yourself.
   D. Come in. We don't trust you, so we have indestructable furniture.
   E. Come in and relax. Enjoy yourself while you wait.
   F. Be yourself; you are okay just the way you are.

Answer: We believe that you have the opportunity to say whatever you wish with the decor of the room and the artifacts placed there. Many people will read the message unconsciously and a few will read it consciously. Either way, they will react to it and set the stage for their contact with you. The communication of the waiting room should be consistent with the style of the staff. An "all business" waiting room should go with an "all business" staff.

Communication is affected by the relative positions of the persons communicating. The transactional positions of "I count" and "I don't count" are important for each person and can be manipulated by furniture. When one person, like the judge in the court room, is seated above the other(s), the setting is a dominant-submissive ("I count—you don't count", or "parent—child") one. The position of the interviewer to the patient may have a profound effect upon some patients.

Question: What position, relative to yourself, do you want to encourage in the patient?

    A. An equal position

    B. A superior, dominant position

    C. An inferior position

Answer: What fits your style? What will help get the current job done? Although the initial position affects the patient, it is not permanent. You can change as the type of treatment changes. As a rule the patient comes to a professional in a dependent position. Hopefully, as time progresses, the patient will grow and become more independent, more responsible for his/her own care. The answer to this question then becomes one of what do you want to encourage at each stage of treatment? Once you decide, manipulate the setting to encourage that behavior on the part of the patient.

Generally, unless the difference in eye level of the two people is more than 6 inches, the two people are in an equal position, communication is on an equal level, and a mutual sharing of responsibility is encouraged. This situation is in marked contrast to that of the patient lying flat on his/her back on a stretcher with the health professional bending over the patient.

Question: What position do you want the patient to be in when you tell him/her what you want him/her to do to take care of the current problem?

Answer: You want the patient in an upright position with feet firmly planted on the floor. Then he/she is in a position to accept responsibly and respond responsibly to what he/she is told.*

------

*See Chapter 8 for elaboration of these ideas.

PART FOUR

PRACTICE INTERVIEWS AND SIMULATIONS

This section of the text is designed to sharpen interviewing skills. Practice interviews provide you with interruptions at critical exchanges. At each of these interruptions you must decide what information he desires, what technique to use, and how to phrase the response. In the interview, "response" refers to the total verbal and nonverbal reaction of the health care professional to the patient. Through a response the interviewer obtains information and guides and supports the patient.

Before working through the following programmed interviews, let us specify four stages in interviewing: (1) the topic is opened: (2) the patient is helped to tell his/her history; (3) the interviewer focuses upon items of special importance; and (4) the interviewer obtains specific information. Although each interview is unique, these four stages generally occur as a repeating sequence for each new topic explored during an interview.

In working through the interviews that follow, you will be asked to select the type of response that is most appropriate at a specific point. As noted in Part I of the manual, several types of responses are useful in more than one stage of exploring a topic. The following summary will aid you in making a selection.

Opening a topic
   Facilitation
   Open-ended question
   Bridging phrase
Assisting the patient's narrative
   Support and reassurance
   Empathy
   Confrontation
   Reflection
   Interpretation
   Silence
   Modified laundry list

Focusing upon a topic
   Confrontation
   Reflection
   Probing
   Interpretation
   Summation
Obtaining specific information
   Direct question
   "Yes" and "no" questions
   Probing
   Problem question
   Laundry list
Closing topic or interview
   Summation
   Prescription for action

INTERVIEW 1

MR. ARNOLD: a medical history

The following interview was conducted by Nathan C. Galloway, M.D.,* an internist, and recorded before a class of second-year medical students. The purpose of the interview was to demonstrate interviewing techniques and to bring out the signs and symptoms of the disease.

The patient was a 55-year-old, medically retired fireman living with his wife on a farm. He was hospitalized for evaluation to decide whether or not he was a candidate for cardiac surgery. When he came to the classroom in a wheel-chair, he was dressed in pajamas and a bathrobe.

Dr.: What sort of trouble are you having?

Pt.: Very severe shortness of breath. I got to where I can't do anything to amount to anything at all. I love to work and I can't. I haven't worked since 1963. I was supposed to be a bed patient until '65. I kinda got off the track. I didn't do as the doctor told me to and now I am behind for it.

Question: Which lead from the patient's speech should one follow?

A. ". . . shortness of breath."
B. ". . . can't do anything. . . "
C. ". . . haven't worked since 1963."
D. ". . . didn't do as the doctor told me to. . . "

Answer: The authors prefer A or B. Our plan is to understand the patient's chief complaint, current symptoms, and current status before going back to the onset of the present illness.

The interviewer chose C, with the evident plan of obtaining information about the onset and the chronologic history of the present illness. Remember, the interviewing

---

*Nathan C. Galloway, M.D., present address, Odessa, Texas.

91

physician is not concerned with treating this patient, but rather with demonstrating the signs and symptoms of the disease.

To focus on the patient's guilt at the opening of an interview, as in D, is usually unproductive. After rapport with the patient has been established, discussion of his guilt may be more therapeutic.

Question: What type of response (that is, facilitation, reflection, direct question) should one make to learn why the patient stopped working in 1963?

Answer: You might make a response of either a reflection or an open-ended question.

Question: Write a response of each type.

Answer: Compare your response with ours.

Reflection: "Haven't worked since 1963," being sure that your vocal inflection does not have any quality of being critical in it.

Open-ended question: See the interviewer's response.

Dr.: What happened in 1963?

Pt.: Well, in '63 is when I had my last attack. And I tried to go back to work after 4 months. It didn't work. I thought I was as good as any man in the department but I wasn't. I work for the fire department. I went back to work and worked about 2 months and found out that I wasn't as good as I thought I was. And so they suggested that I could get my pension.

Question: Where should one go from here? What information do you want? The patient has presented the following phrases, choose one upon which to have him focus.

A. ". . . my last attack."
B. ". . . tried to go back to work. . . . "
C. ". . . work for the fire department."
D. ". . . could get my pension."

Answer: Because of his last response, the interviewer is committed to finding out about the onset of the illness, A. The key word *last* in "my last attack" signals that the illness began at an earlier time. The interviewer focused upon this. When a physician has information about the patient's present symptoms, it is easier for him to spot the early symptoms that pinpoint the onset of the illness. This is why the authors preferred A or B at the onset of the interview.

B offers an opening for discussing the symptoms and history of illness after his attack in 1963. The history obtained from the 1963 starting point, in the middle of the illness, will suffer from the lack of a logical time sequence. The patient and physician will be able to understand each other with less confusion if the data-gathering is accomplished along a logical pathway.

C and D will not lead directly to establishing information about the patient's illness. These topics lead into the social history that is usually obtained after the information about the organic components of the illness has been noted.

Question: To learn about the onset of this man's illness, what type of response would you make?

Answer: You might make a response of any of the following types: reflection, confrontation, open-ended question (or statement), or facilitation.

Question: Make up a reflection, confrontation, open-ended question (or statement), and facilitation that will lead to the onset of the patient's illness.

Answer: Compare your responses with ours.
A. Reflection: "1963 was your *last* attack."
B. Confrontation: *"Last* attack!"
C. Open-ended statement: "I see. Tell me about your first attack."
D. Facilitation: "Your trouble began before 1963."

The interviewer combined a reflection with a direct question, which, as expected, received a short answer.

Dr.: Now, you say your last attack was in '63. When was your first one?
Pt.: 1957.
Dr.: And what happened in 1957?
Pt.: Well, I was fishing and I had my boat pulled up in some snags so it would not float downstream. All of a sudden a pain hit me in the chest. I was tying up the front end of the boat. The pain hit me in the chest and my left arm, not in my shoulder. It wasn't a sharp pain; it was a dull ache and I tried to reel in my line and untie. I couldn't do that so I did untie the boat and cut my line. Then I started passing out. I was by myself on the river and there wasn't another boat around so I floated down the river about seven miles. At times I'd come to and times I'd pass out.
Dr.: Were you hurting for a long time?

Pt.: When I was conscious I was hurting, yes. I moored into the boat dock down there. Two men were up on the bank, but they couldn't see me. My throat swelled shut. I couldn't holler at them, and when I felt as if I was going to pass out, I laid down in the boat to keep from falling out. Finally one of them came down. I motioned to him "my heart" and he called his friend down. They carried me up on the bank and called the fire department. They took me directly to the hospital.

Dr.: Where was that?

Pt.: St. Mary's Hospital. And I spent 3 weeks in the hospital.

Dr.: Who did you doctor with then?

Comment: The last two direct questions by the physician orient the patient's history geographically, and they establish information needed to obtain past medical records. One may question whether this interruption of the patient's story is justified. A ward secretary can obtain this information when it is needed, or it can be ascertained from a history form filled out by the patient. The physician does not usually need the name of the previous physician to understand either the illness or his patient. As you will see, this interruption did not affect the flow of information from this patient, but it will affect the flow of information in many interviews. This patient's responsiveness may be partly the result of this physician's ability to phrase questions in the patient's vernacular, that is, "Who did you *doctor with* then?"

Pt.: I started out with Dr. A. He was our family doctor. He referred me to a heart specialist, Dr. B. I stayed in the hospital 3 weeks, then went home and stayed in bed for better than 2 months. At the beginning of the fourth month I got up and began getting a little exercise. After the fourth month I thought I was strong enough to go back to work. I did go back to work but found out that I wasn't strong enough.

Question: How would you learn more about what happened when the patient went back to work? What kind of response would you make?

Answer: You might respond with any of the following types: reflection, facilitation, summation, or open-ended question.

Question: Make up a response to the patient for each of the following:

    A. Reflection
    B. Facilitation
    C. Summation
    D. Open-ended question

Answer: Compare your response with ours.
  A. Reflection: "You weren't strong enough!"
  B. Facilitation: "Uh huh!"
  C. Summation: "After 4 months you weren't strong enough."
  D. Open-ended question: "What did you notice?" *or* "What happened?"

Note: A combination of a reflection and an open-ended question is often effective, that is, "You found out! In what way?" Any of these responses are effective. The interviewer's response is effective, but it requires a second question before the patient returns to his earlier free flow of information.

Dr.: How did you know?
Pt.: The first fire.
Dr.: What happened?
Pt.: I couldn't do what I thought I could do. I didn't have the strength. I don't have the strength in my left arm and can't control it too well. When I go to do something, almost anything at all, lifting any weight or anything fast, I have to stop and take a nitroglycerin.
Dr.: It didn't work, or it hurt?
Pt.: It hurt, and when it hurts you don't work.

Question: What does *it* refer to?
  A. Left arm
  B. Chest
  C. Heart
  D. Nitroglycerin

Answer: A and C as you will see from the interview. Pronouns frequently need clarification. Many times the patient and physician are talking about two different topics because of confusion over pronouns. Don't be afraid to say, "I don't know what you mean by it (he, she)." You may even introduce an ambiguous pronoun to get the patient to specify or clarify a point of information.

Question: Make up a response to clarify this ambiguous use of *it*.

Answer: Did you use a laundry-list question? This is a natural place for one. Compare your response with our responses. "I don't know what you mean by 'it hurt'." *or* "It hurt! Do you mean that the hurting was in your arm, chest, or where?"

Dr.: It hurt! Do you mean that the hurting was in your chest, arm, or where?
Pt.: Heart and arm.
Dr.: In your chest, too?

Pt.: No, just in the heart part. It felt like you might just stick an ice pick in there and whirl it around.

Dr.: You told us the first pain was a dull ache, but now this pain is sharp or what?

Pt.: It's still a dull pain in the arm, but it's a very sharp pain in the heart.

Dr.: It's sharp there?

Pt.: Yes.

Dr.: Could you point to where it is on your chest?

Pt.: Yes, right here (pointing to an area about the size of a silver dollar).

Dr.: How long does it usually last when you have it?

Pt.: It lasts until I take enough nitros to knock it and at first I'd time it. I'd take one nitro and it would take 40 seconds to knock it. Now it gets to where I take three nitros and it takes a minute and 20 seconds.

Question: How would you establish the severity of the pain in this patient? Make up a response to the patient.

Answer: Methods range from simply asking, "How bad is the pain?" to finding out what behavior occurs with the pain. From this latter data one can infer how severe the pain is (that is, does it require the patient to stop what he is doing).

Dr.: Now have you ever had any pain worse than that?

Pt.: No, never.

Dr.: Have you ever had a broken bone?

Pt.: Yes.

Dr.: How does the heart pain compare with the pain of the broken bone?

Pt.: That felt good. I sawed my leg with a chain saw and they put twenty seven stitches in it. I sawed into some bone and it felt good compared to this.

Question: Since information about the severity of the symptoms has been obtained, the next point of focus concerns the behavior associated with the symptoms, specifically, whether or not the symptoms come on at rest. Should one ask directly about this? Or is some bridging phrase of comment needed?

Answer: A bridging comment is needed.

Question: Make up a bridging comment and compare it with the one used by the interviewer.

Dr.: Now you say when you start hurrying around or lifting is the time you have this pain. Do you ever have this pain when you're just lying around?

Pt.: I did for awhile, it would come on about 2 o'clock in the morning.

Dr.: About 2 o'clock in the morning? (A reflection.)

Pt.: Yes, about 2 o'clock in the morning and the doctor added another one of the pills I was taking at bedtime.

Dr.: Was that a two-toned green pill?

Pt.: Right. And since that time I don't have any more pain at night.

> **Comment:** Sufficient data has been gained about this topic. Note how the bridging phrase is used to make a logical lead into the next topic.

Dr.: After your first attack, when you got out of the hospital, what sort of medicines were you taking?

Pt.: I can't tell you for sure. I don't remember. I was taking nitros, and a two-toned green pill, and a nerve capsule.

Dr.: Were you getting prothrombin times then?

> **Comment:** Patients receiving anticoagulant therapy are informed about the therapy and must have their blood checked periodically for prothrombin time (coagulation time). Thus, it is not unusual for this patient to recognize this medical term.

Pt.: Yes, I still go in every month for a check on that. (Pause.) And in '62 I had another heart attack.

Dr.: Was that the second one.

Pt.: Yes, that was the second one.

> **Question:** What information should one now seek?
>
> A. Details of the patient's second attack.
> B. History of interval between attacks.
> C. Further details about prothrombin time.

> **Answer:** B. Our reason for not selecting A is that gathering information about the patient's second attack may make it more difficult to later obtain the interval (between attacks) history. It may also make it more difficult to piece the information together. However, the patient jumped to this topic and is ready to discuss it.
>
> Further data about the patient's prothrombin time, C, will serve little useful purpose in diagnosis and treatment. He probably does not know the details a physician needs for planning further therapy. For this information the physician obtains the patient's past medical record.

> **Question:** What type of response would you use to obtain the interval history?

> **Answer:** Any of the following types may be effective: open-ended question, bridging phrase followed by an open-ended question, or summation.

> **Question:** Make up a response of each type.

Answer: Open-ended question: "What happened between '57 and '62?"

Bridging phrase followed by an open-ended question: "Let's go back a minute first. Tell me how things were between '57 and '62." *or* "I see, but first, how were you between attacks?"

Summation: (See below.)

Dr.:   Now, you had an attack in '57 and went back to work in about 4 months?

Pt.:   Yes.

Dr.:   And you were having pain when you really had to hurry?

Pt.:   That's right. When we weren't at a fire, I wouldn't have to take any nitros.

Dr.:   Was there anything around the house that seemed to cause you to have pain?

Pt.:   I couldn't cut grass and I still can't.

Dr.:   And what about intercourse?

Pt.:   Very much so. I would take three nitros before I started and three when I finished and if I was lucky I would get by on that.

Question: This information gives one a fair idea of the patient's cardiac status between attacks. Now, how does one return to the second attack and get information about it? Make up a response.

Answer: Compare your response with the interviewer's.

Dr.:   And then in '62 you had another attack. What were you doing when this one came on?

Pt.:   I was fishing.

Dr.:   You were still working then?

Pt.:   Yes.

Dr.:   What was the attack like?

Pt.:   It was the same thing only it wasn't quite as great. It wasn't quite as hard a pain, but it was the same.

Dr.:   And then!

Pt.:   When the pain hits, you stop whatever you're doing. If it's a pretty hard one, you lie down. It doesn't make any difference whether you're in some snow or mud, you lie down.

Dr.:   That's just what you need to do.

Pt.:   It's something to get rid of it quicker. I don't know why it is, but lying down seems to have a quicker effect of the nitros, so that's what you do.

Dr.:   What do you do after you've taken the nitros in an attack and they don't help?

Pt.:   You keep taking more.

Dr.:   Do you stay real still or do you try to shake it off?

Pt.:   No, you stay real still and take deep breaths, just as deep as you can get them. I was advised against taking more than three nitros, but I have taken as high as eleven and if it hurt bad enough I guess I would take twenty five.

Question: How should one get to the information about the details of the second attack? What type of a response should one make?

    A.   Direct question
    B.   Empathic
    C.   Open-ended question
    D.   Summation followed by an open-ended question

Answer: We prefer B, C, or D.

Question: Make up a response of each type and compare them with ours.

Answer:
    A.   Direct question: See below and note the short answer this patient gave to the question.
    B.   Empathic: "The second attack was a rough experience," *or* "The pain of an attack can be pretty great."
    C.   Open-ended question: "What happened after the second attack?"
    D.   Summation and open-ended question: "With the attack you lay down. Then what happened?"

Dr.: Now after this second attack how long were you in the hospital?
Pt.: I was in the hospital about 2½ weeks with the second one.

Comment: The direct question has value in obtaining concise information quickly. In a patient who rambles, direct questions are needed early in the exploration of a topic to obtain the most useful information in the time allotted.

Dr.: Two and one-half weeks. It didn't seem to be quite as bad as the first one?

Comment: Note how responsive this patient is to the interviewer's demonstration of understanding of what he had said.

Pt.: No, and then I went home and stayed in bed quite awhile, for about the same period of time. In 4 months I went back to work again. I seemed to get over those two all right. But, I couldn't do the job that I was supposed to do, although I had good enough buddies working with me. They carried me through.
Dr.: Tell me what you mean, you "couldn't do the job you were supposed to do."

Pt.: Well, people think that when you work for the fire department you sleep and eat and play cards. You do to a certain extent and the work is very easy around the fire station. But, when the alarm goes off you are working under the most extreme conditions there are. You work just as hard and just as fast as you can work. You carry heavier loads than you would ordinarily carry. A hose for instance is a two-man job, but if there isn't another man there you just pick it up and go on with it. Those are the things I could not do.

Question: When hearing a patient present this example, one wants to know just what symptoms he had when he would "go on with it." What type of response would you make?

Answer: Open-ended question.

Question: What would be wrong with using a direct question or a laundry-list question in this situation?

Answer: Both types of response will suggest symptoms to the patient, that is, "Did you have pain in your heart, pain in your arm, shortness of breath, or flushing of your face?" *or* "Did you have pain in your heart?"

Question: Make up an open-ended question.

Answer: Compare your response with the interviewer's.

Dr.: What did you notice when you were "working under extreme conditions?"
Pt.: I had angina and was short of breath.
Dr.: Were you having as much angina after the second attack?
Pt.: Yes, about the same. Month by month, after I went back to work for about 6 months, I could tell I was getting a little better all along. I still didn't follow my doctor's orders. I mean, he told me to take it easy and on my days off to get some rest; but I like to work.
Dr.: There are things to be done around the house, aren't there?
Pt.: Yes, and other places, too. In other words, I worked on my days off and made a little extra money. I did things I shouldn't do and should have gotten more rest. The doctor didn't know I was doing them so that's how things turn out.

Question: The patient has just expressed the feeling that he is to blame for his present condition. One might interpret this as a request for support and reassurance—a request for being excused from responsibility—assurance that his illness would have continued whether he worked or rested. What type of response would you make in this situation?

Answer: Confrontation.

Question: Indicate what would be wrong with a statement such as, "Well, no one knows what might have been, but you did what you thought you could do."

Answer: Such a statement may or may not be true. But it does block the feeling from further discussion. Hasty reassurance is usually felt as a rebuff or rejection by the patient. It also implies that he did not do more than he should have done. This response would increase his guilt if he had been more active than he should have.

Question: How would you phrase a confrontation?

Answer: Compare your confrontation with ours.

"Sounds like you blame yourself for this."
"Sounds like you are being pretty hard on yourself."
"You seem to blame yourself for this."
"You just couldn't be inactive?"

Note: An alternate course of action was taken in the interview. The feeling was sidestepped and the patient's attention was redirected to the account of his illness. Both the patient's self-blame and a further account of his illness will have to be discussed before the patient can be successfully treated. The topic to be examined first is the interviewer's choice.

Dr.: And then when did you have your third attack?
Pt.: I had my third attack in '63.
Dr.: How did this one come on?
Pt.: It came on the same way. I was raising a trotline and when it hit, my wife was in the boat.
Dr.: How long did it take to know that it wasn't just angina?
Pt.: Right away.
Dr.: You mean you know within just a minute?
Pt.: Within seconds.
Dr.: It was different from the angina?
Pt.: Yes.
Dr.: Aside from the intensity, was there anything else different?
Pt.: No. It was just harder.
Dr.: And there's no question in your mind that you can tell whether it was angina or a heart attack?

Question: What is wrong with the doctor's last question as written?

Answer: The question as phrased places the patient on the defensive by challenging his last statements.

Question: Rephrase the question so that it does not provoke defensiveness in the patient.

Answer: "When the pain began, did you have any question whether it was angina or a heart attack?" *or* "Is there any question in your mind that you can tell whether it was angina or a heart attack?"

Pt.: No. (Pause.) That was the lightest attack of them all. It was about 30 minutes until we were able to get into town.

Dr.: The pain lasted about 30 minutes?

Pt.: Yes, it let up enough that I could get on into the stationwagon and into town with my wife. I never could kick any part of that last heart attack. I went back to work and I worked about 2 months. We had a fire and I was down there about 6 hours. I always carried from twenty five to forty nitros in a little container. I don't know for sure how many I had, but I ran out of nitros. I took the chief's car up to a drugstore. I got fifty more and when I got back to the station, I had about six or eight of them left. I must have taken between sixty and seventy. The next day was my day to see my doctor and we talked about the fire. He asked me how I got along down there and I said "fine." He asked me how many nitros I took and that time I told him the truth. The next day the chief came down to the station and told me I could get my retirement if I wanted. I didn't want to take it, but I knew I was just taking the place of a good man down there, so I took my retirement and I got out.

Dr.: Now, what have you been doing since then?

Pt.: That was when I was supposed to go home and get my exercise by going from the chair to the bed and the bed to the chair. That was the last part of '63. It was just before Christmas in '65 when they told me I could get up and start walking the length of our house five times a day. But in the meantime I got awfully irritable and nervous and everything. I love children but I couldn't be around them very long. They would run up and pick flowers or ring the doorbell. It was pretty rough. I told my wife we had to get out of town. We moved eleven miles out of town. We bought a place with a lake out there. I was still supposed to be in bed, but instead of doing that I was out cutting brush—I mean not very much, I'd work maybe 3 minutes. I had a Homelite chain saw. I'd work for 3 minutes then I'd sit down and rest for 10 minutes.

Dr.: Did your disposition get better?

Pt.: No.

Dr.: And your pain?

Pt.: It kept getting worse and that's the reason I'm here now because I didn't have enough sense to listen the first time.

Comment: This is the third time the patient has alluded to feelings of guilt. The patient's statement is an opening to explore his feelings.

Question: Make up a response that will probe his feelings related to "didn't have enough sense to listen the first time."

Answer: Several approaches might be equally effective with this patient.

Facilitation: "How is that?" *or* "How do you see it?"

Reflection: "You didn't have enough sense?" *or* "That's the reason you are here?"

Confrontation: "You really feel it is your fault?" This can be said so that it challenges or casts some doubt upon the patient's feeling, or it could be phrased, "Sounds like you feel rather guilty."

Empathic: "Those are not comfortable feelings to live with." *or* "You see your situation differently now."

Dr.: How do you see it?
Pt.: I knew at the time that I was doing more than I should, but I couldn't stop. I was irritable and nervous, just seemed as if I couldn't stand it in the house. It got to where everything I did caused me pain or shortness of breath.
Dr.: At those times you think a lot about life.
Pt.: Yes, you read the Bible, you pray, and you try to find a way.

Question: A physician wants to know how depressed the patient has been. Make up a response which will elicit this information.

Answer: Compare your response with the interviewer's.

Dr.: How low would your feelings get when you would think like that?
Pt.: Pretty low.

Question: The patient has indicated by his answer that he has been depressed at times. One wants to know if he is or has been considering suicide. Make up a response which will shed light on this topic.

Answer: Compare your response with ours.
"Have you ever felt so low that you have thought about hurting yourself?" *or* "Have you ever felt that life is not worth living?"

Also note the interviewer's response.

Dr.: Ever wonder about ending it all?
Pt.: Yes, many times.
Dr.: What would happen then?
Pt.: Oh, sometimes I would feel that way for days. I never tried anything, but I thought a lot about it.

Question: One wants to know what his thoughts were to understand just how serious his depression was. Make up a response and compare it with the interviewer's.

Dr.: Like what?
Pt.: Once I thought of taking my gun and ending it all, so I asked my wife

to give my gun to the neighbor. She did and never seemed to know why. I told her I couldn't use it and my neighbor liked to hunt. That was the only time the thoughts got to me.

Comment: This gives one an understanding of this patient's degree of depression in the past and how he reacted to it. The question is, "How depressed is he now?" Following the frank discussion that just preceded, one can ask directly about the patient's present feelings.

Dr.: How have you felt about it lately?

Pt.: With this possible operation, I have not thought about it much. I am just anxious for them to tell me whether or not they will operate.

Question: It seems obvious that the patient has hope if an operation takes place, but if the doctors decide not to operate, how will he react? We believe this topic should be discussed. Make up a response which will elicit the information.

Answer: Compare your response with the following:

a. "There is still some doubt whether or not they will operate?"
    Follow up this opening with the question, "If they do not operate, what then?"

b. "You have some concern that they will not operate!"
    "It's not easy waiting to learn of their decision."
    Follow the patient's reply with, "If they do not operate, what then?"

Also note the interviewer's response.

Dr.: And if they do not operate?

Pt.: That wouldn't be easy to take, but I will have to face it. I'll just have to do what they tell me to.

Dr.: Do you think these thoughts will return?

Pt.: Yes, but I have learned not to let them bother me. I just read something or think about something else.

Question: His method of handling depression sounds reasonable as far as he has gone. But what if he cannot "read something, or think about something else?" One needs to know his next line of defense against depression. Make up a response to learn about his next steps to fight depression and compare it with the interviewer's.

Dr.: What will you do if you cannot shake off the thoughts?

Pt.: Well, I have been able to talk to Dr. A. about them and he will help me if I need the help.

Comment: This sequence leaves the patient with the feeling that the physician understands and is interested in him. The physician has an understanding of the patient's level of, and reactions to, depression. Note the bridging phrase to return to the remaining information needed about the present illness.

Dr.: Very good. Now I would like to learn a little more about how you were since 1965. Were you continuing to have the angina right along?

Pt.: Yes.

Dr.: Were you having any difficulty with shortness of breath when you exerted yourself?

Pt.: Yes.

Dr.: When did you begin to notice it?

Pt.: I just cannot say. It gradually got worse and worse to the point where I couldn't walk down to the lake without having to stop and rest. It was only about three-quarters of a block from the house.

Dr.: Did you have to stop even when you were going downhill?

Pt.: I could go downhill without stopping, but I'd have to stop twice on the way back up.

Question: At this point the interviewer needs to know about other symptoms of congestive heart failure, specifically, whether or not the patient's feet have swollen. What type of response should one use to obtain this information?

Answer: Direct question.

Question: Make up a direct question and compare it with the interviewer's response.

Dr.: Have you had any swelling of your feet?

Pt.: No.

Dr.: What medicines are you on at this time?

Pt.: I'm on this two-tone green, and digoxin, and Diuril, and Coumadin, and—well, there's fourteen different kinds in all.

Dr.: That is quite a lot. (Pause.) I was wondering, did you have any trouble with your heart when you sawed into your leg?

Pt.: No. Didn't have any angina then. (Pause.) I don't get upset. You can tell me whatever you want to, say what you want to, or do what you want to. You cannot make me angry even if you tried. If you did make me angry, I would suffer for 3 days with angina. So you cannot make me angry even if you try. I just get my mind on something else.

Dr.: When you get angry you have more angina?

Pt.: Yes.

Dr.: I see. Now I have asked you a number of questions. Do you have any questions you wish to ask me?

Pt.: (Pause, thoughtfully.) No.

Dr.: Mr. Arnold, you have given us a clear picture of your illness and your treatment. Now your job is to work with your doctor to learn whether or not an operation will be of help to you.

Pt.: That's right.

Dr.: I wish to thank you for letting me interview you today. I will wheel you back to your room now.

Pt.: Okay.

INTERVIEW 2

MRS. KING: a marital history

The following recorded interview occurred as part of an out-patient evaluation by Robert E. Froelich, M.D.* The patient is a 27-year-old white nurse who has been married 5 years and who is the mother of two children (3 years and 10 months). She is coming to the physician because of weight loss. After several minutes of the interview, during which the patient describes her present symptoms of weight loss, anorexia, tiredness, and depression, the following exchange takes place. (The physician began to actively explore the patient's marital relationship to further understand her symptoms.)

Dr.: What is the relationship between you and your husband?

Pt.: There is absolutely no communication between us at all. I mean even as far as discussion. I find Bill very difficult to discuss any particular problem with, at all. He is very narrow minded in his viewpoint, or closed to any suggestion. It is very difficult to approach him in any way.

Dr.: And this has gone on now for how long, would you say?

Pt.: Oh, I would say like this for about a year. A little over a year.

Dr.: Uh huh, and during this time you haven't been able to talk at all? (Pause.) Is it that you haven't been able to talk or you haven't been able to agree?

Pt.: That's a good question. Because it seems like even from the beginning of our marriage it has been difficult to discuss anything with Bill. I mean that he finds it very difficult to accept anybody else's ideas or opinions.

Dr.: Uh huh, what is he like when he is at home?

Pt.: Tired, and he usually comes in and flops down and watches TV or reads the paper or a magazine. He is the type of person that doesn't do much after he comes home. He reads the paper and that is about it. That and TV.

Dr.: Are there any activities that you do together?

Pt.: No, not wholeheartedly, no. His hobby is road racing, which I just go along with because he is interested in it. There are few outings that the

---

*University of Alabama in Huntsville.

whole family can participate in together. I am active in church work and he never goes to church. He is active in Masonic work and I can't be a part of that. So I would say that we have no existing activity together.

Dr.: Well, with this sort of each going his own way, like two students sharing a house—

Pt.: (Interrupting.) That is about it. (The patient might have continued had the physician not insisted upon completing his question.)

Dr.: What does this do to marital relations, sexual relations?

Pt.: It dampens them completely, because you aren't communicating anything, and as you say, we are both living separate lives almost.

Dr.: So there is little or no sexual contact now?

Pt.: There is little.

Dr.: And what about before this past year?

Pt.: It seems like each year it gets less and less. From my viewpoint it is because there is a lack of communication, and, along with this, he has little interest in home life.

Question: What type of response would you use to learn of the patient's reaction to sexual relations (enjoys, disquieted by, or what)?

Answer: Direct question (if you are careful not to suggest an answer)
Laundry-list question
Open-ended question

Question: Make up a response of each type.

Answer: Direct question: "Do you look forward to having relations?"

Laundry-list question: see the interviewer's response

Open-ended question: "What is your reaction to having sexual relations?"

Dr.: When you do have relations, it is something that is enjoyable, something that is tolerated, or something that is *comme ci, comme ca,* or what?

Pt.: Well, I would say for me they are tolerated right now.

Dr.: And for him?

Pt.: I don't know, but I would say tolerated at this point.

Comment: Another criterion for understanding how two people are relating to one another involves knowing who initates sexual activity.

Question: How would you inquire? Make up a response.

Answer: See interviewer's response.

Dr.: Who initiates the act?

Pt.:   I would say both, but most generally he initiates it.
Dr.:   How does that compare with early in your marriage?
Pt.:   The exact opposite.

> **Question:**   Do you know what the patient means? Does she mean that she initiated sexual relations early in the marriage? Make up a response to clarify her last reply.

> **Answer:**   "The exact opposite?" (A reflection.)
> "I don't understand, opposite."
> "I don't follow."
>
> See interviewer's response.

Dr.:   By that you mean—
Pt.:   They were very frequent at first. (Pause.)
Dr.:   And?
Pt.:   And we both enjoyed them and most generally he initiated it.
Dr.:   How long were you married when your first child arrived?

> **Comment:**   This seeming change of topic occurred because the physician wished to learn whether the pregnancy was a major factor in altering the couple's relationship.

Pt.:   Two years.
Dr.:   Was there any change, after that, in your relations?
Pt.:   Not particularly.

> **Comment:**   The patient reports that she was about to leave her husband just before she learned that she was pregnant with her second child. She decided that it would be too hard to live alone with two children and decided to stay with her husband. Later in the interview during the review of systems, the following exchange took place:

Dr.:   What are your menstrual periods like now?
Pt.:   Let's see, my periods are about 30 or 32 days apart.
Dr.:   And the flow?
Pt.:   Is very light.
Dr.:   And a period lasts how long?
Pt.:   Oh, about 4 days.
Dr.:   You started having periods at what age?
Pt.:   Thirteen years.
Dr.:   How old were you when you had your first pregnancy?
Pt.:   I was 20.

> **Question:**   A little quick addition indicated that the patient was 22 years old when she was married. How do you learn about this first pregnancy? Make up your response.

> **Answer:**   "Were you married at the time?" (Because of social conventions, this question may place undue stress on the patient; and it may suggest that you will be judgmental.)

"That was before your present marriage?" (The judgmental quality of this question is not as strong; in fact, if it is said matter of factly, it can be a neutral clarification.)

Dr.: Was that before your present marriage?
Pt.: Yes.

Question: What is the information you need about this pregnancy to understand the patient's present life adjustment?

Answer: The circumstances that led up to the pregnancy, its outcome (marriage, abortion, delivery, and adoption) and how the patient views the event after 7 years.

Question: Make up a response, to the patient, to learn of the circumstances and compare it with the interviewer's response.

Dr.: What were the circumstances?
Pt.: The father of the child was a guy I had been going with off and on for about a year. And the night before, I went home. (Pause.) This was in January before I was to be graduated from nurses' training in June. (Tears come to the patient's eyes.) Our house was over a mile from the hospital. I walked home as I didn't have any money. I went home to see if Daddy would give me any money. I don't remember exactly what happened, but Daddy and I were doing the dishes and we were talking. He was wanting to know what I was going to do after I was graduated. I told him that I wanted to go on to school if I could get enough money for tuition. He asked me how much I thought I would need. I told him that I would probably need about three or four hundred dollars. Norma, my stepmother, walked in about then and said that they weren't about to help me get money for tuition. I turned around and said back to her that I didn't think that I would call back to her for help. That was the first time I had ever talked back to her. (Pause.) She and Daddy got into a big fight, which lasted the rest of the evening. I don't remember all that the fight was about, but I do remember vividly that I had never felt so all alone. (Pause.) Anyway, I had a date with this fellow the next night. We went out to dinner and then went dancing. I started drinking, and I guess that was the first time in my life that I had ever been drunk. Things just went too far. I never saw him after that. I told him that I didn't want to see him again.
Dr.: You told him that the next day?
Pt.: I told him that night.

Question: Make up a response to explore the patient's feelings toward the father of the child.

Answer: Compare your response with the interviewer's response.

Dr.: But until then you had a good opinion of him?
Pt.: Oh, I liked him. I didn't know too much about him. He was a likable

fellow. He must have come from a very wealthy family. He sold insurance. I never thought much about it at the time, but he was driving a new Cadillac with a gold grill, which meant nothing to me then. He had asked me many times to marry him, but I just laughed it off.

Dr.: He was several years older?

Pt.: Yes, I don't know exactly how much older he was. I was never really sure about his age.

Question: What information do you now desire?

Answer: What was the outcome of the pregnancy?

Question: Make up a response and compare it with the interviewer's response.

Dr.: What was the pregnancy like?

Pt.: I guess it was 42 days before graduation, we had our school physical exams. The doctor felt my enlarged uterus. He said that he would have to tell the director of nurses. I begged him not to tell her because I knew I would be kicked out. But he said that he would talk to her, and surprisingly enough, I wasn't. I didn't know what I would do and she arranged for me to work in another hospital. My family didn't know that I was pregnant. After graduation and state boards, I started to work right away. It was a very rough start because they didn't pay but once a month. I worked straight through, including extra shifts, up until the day before the baby was born and started back 9 days later. I worked on about a month.

Question: This history is presented hesitantly, between tears and with strong feeling. How should you respond?

Answer: Some show of understanding, empathy, or support is in order.

Question: Make up a response that would show understanding, support, or empathy.

Answer: Compare your responses with these.

"That must not have been easy without a family's support."

"That was a lot for a 20-year-old to go through alone."

See the interviewer's response.

Dr.: Sounds like you succeeded in this difficult situation with no help from home. What about the decision regarding the future of the child? Was this made for you, were you a part of the decision making, or what?

Pt.: No, I made the decision, I talked to numerous people about it, I had decided that it was best to give the child up.

Dr.: How do you feel about it today?

Pt.: I guess I still wonder. But at the time it seemed that was the most difficult thing I had ever done in my life, to turn around and walk away from my baby.

> **Comment:** At this point the interviewer has the choice between exploring the feeling further or changing the focus to less emotionally charged factual material. In therapy the feeling would be pursued with either a reflection or an empathic response. In the data-gathering interview the topic can be changed as follows.

Dr.: Was it a boy or girl?

Pt.: It was a girl.

Dr.: She is how old now?

Pt.: She will be 7 this year.

Dr.: Do you know anything about who adopted her?

Pt.: No, I have no idea.

Dr.: No idea?

Pt.: No idea, but I think that the Sisters either had a nice family picked out or another time I heard that the doctor who delivered me wanted her, but I don't know where she went. I never tried to find out.

> **Question:** Make up a response to learn how the patient now views this pregnancy. Compare your response with the interviewer's.

Dr.: Is this something that crosses your mind now? Or does this happen only when someone mentions it?

Pt.: It is virtually impossible for me to answer because now I don't know if it would cross my mind every so often or not. But Bill can be so psychologically cruel and he keeps throwing it up to me.

Dr.: Then, you told Bill about the child?

Pt.: Yes.

> **Comment:** Physicians sometimes believe that special techniques are needed to explore a patient's sexual feeling and behavior. But, as just demonstrated, the techniques learned earlier in this manual can explore these topics effectively.
>
> Knowledge of a patient's sexual behavior may help the physician understand the patient's more private or guarded feelings that may not be evident from other interpersonal information. The knowledge of sexual behavior will help the physician to formulate his diagnosis and treatment plan.
>
> Sexual behavior between two people is an extension of their daily interpersonal interactions. During the sexual act any feelings known to man, from tenderness to sadism, may be expressed.

MR. DEVOE: a fearful patient

A 27-year-old, white, right-handed male, Mr. Joe Devoe, has a history of a broken arm (compound fracture) resulting from an occupational accident in a meat-packing plant 4 months ago. The fracture was of the right humerus with some damage to the radial nerve. The patient has been seeing you in follow-up. You are, then, fairly familiar with his condition. He is currently out of work because of numbness in his hand, along with complaints that he is unable to work. He states that his hand "does not work as well as it used to."

1. *Dr.:* Mr. Devoe, what is the trouble today?
    Pt.: You know, Doc, I still have trouble with this hand of mine—I still can't use it too well.

Instructions: Choose the response you prefer, then skip to the answer for that response. If you select the preferred response, you will continue with the interview directly. If you select a wrong or less preferred response, you will be directed to "try again" or directed to the preferred response. Some readers prefer to read all the comments to the wrong responses.

> *Dr.:*   A. You're still having trouble?
> B. Where's it bothering you now?
> C. What can't you do with your hand?
> D. What can you do with your hand?

Answer A: *Dr.:* You're still having trouble?
Pt.: Yes, it's about the same every day—I pick up some then I get worse. Don't know what it is.

> **Note:** This reflection may convey the meaning to the patient that you are not happy to see him or that you didn't expect to see him again. Happily for you the patient has overlooked this, at least superficially.

Dr.: In what way does it pick up, then get worse?
Pt.: Well, I'll get so I can use it fairly well, then it will get to where I can't use it again.

Dr.: How's that?
Pt.: I just seem to lose use of it for a time, can't seem to get it to do what I want it to do.
Dr.: How does your hand feel then?
Pt.: Well, it feels numb, like when you hold a piece of frozen meat in your hand too long, you know?
(Skip to No. 2.)

Answer B: Dr.: Where's it bothering you now?
Pt.: Oh, you know, the usual place, my right hand.

> Note: You have asked a question that is too specific. Let the patient pick his own sector. Respect his judgment on what is significant. Try again.

Answer C: Dr.: What can't you do with your hand?
Pt.: There are lots of things that I cannot do with it—such as button my shirt, write very well, and things like that.

> Note: You lead the patient strongly toward the manifest complaint. You are interested in the manifest complaint, but with a potential disability case on your hands, you are also interested in the latent content. Try again.

Answer D: Dr.: What can you do with your hand?
Pt.: Well, I can eat all right and write some—I can't button my clothes too well or do much close work.
Dr.: Does it get better?
Pt.: It will stop feeling frozen, and I can start using it a little more, but pretty soon I just seem to lose use of it for a time, can't seem to get it to do what I want it to do. It feels numb, like when you hold a piece of frozen meat too long, you know?

> Note: You have asked a question about positive aspects of the patient's condition, rather than negative ones. This should encourage the patient to limit his discussion to the positives, that is, his *abilities*, rather than his *disabilities*. You may have also noted that it was only a short period of time until he was again relating to the negative (to response A).

2. Comment: At this interview you have the report from the hospital to which the patient has reported recently for physical therapy and to have the extent of nerve involvement at the fracture site determined. The hospital reports that their findings are essentially negative. They feel that the nervous tissue has returned to normal. Impairment, at any rate, is slight. The numbness does not follow the radial nerve distribution, but rather it follows ego boundaries (culturally determined body segments, that is, finger, hand, wrist, forearm).

Pt.: Well, it feels numb, like when you hold a piece of frozen meat in your hand too long, you know!

Dr.: A. Mr. Devoe, the report I have been given states that you should have good control by now. Are you sure you are not imagining this?

B. When do you notice this numbness or loss of feeling?

Answer A: *Dr.:* Mr. Devoe, the report I have been given states that you should have good control by now. Are you sure you are not imagining this?

Pt.: No, Doc, it's just as real as the nose on my face. I swear I'm not imagining this.

Note: He's not imagining anything—in fact, there may be some numbness in the limb. The lab reports didn't entirely exclude this possibility. How can you tell anyone else what they feel? Sensations are private information. Try again.

Answer B: *Dr.:* When do you notice this numbness or loss of feeling?

Pt.: Oh, I notice it when I first get up and it carries on throughout the day.

Note: The question you just asked was acceptable. A better question, however, might have been "How do you notice this numbness?" After all, this patient has been in to see you several times for the same complaint. What you would like to know now is, "has the condition changed remarkably and how does the patient understand it?" You need specific examples to understand this patient. (Continue to No. 3.)

3. *Dr.:* And how does it affect your life?

Pt.: Oh, it ruins my life. I can't do any work or anything.

Dr.: And have you tried to go back to work?

Pt.: Yes, for a couple of days, but my hand was still bad and it's not getting any better.

Dr.: A. And you feel it is foolish to try so hard when you seem to improve so little?

B. How can you expect to get better with an attitude like that?

C. Since you aren't working, how are you getting along?

D. How do you plan to get along if it doesn't get any better?

E. Well, just what can you do?

Answer A: *Dr.:* And you feel it is foolish to try so hard when you seem to improve so little?

            Pt.: Oh, Doc—I don't mind trying to get my hand back in shape; I want it to get better. That's why I came to you.

            Note: He would like to deny it. He realizes the social unacceptability of not working. He would like, in any case, to give you the picture of an ideal, cooperative patient. He knows the role well. Note that you have challenged him. Try again.

Answer B: *Dr.:* How can you expect to get better with an attitude like that?

            Pt.: It's not my attitude I came in to see you about doctor, it's my hand.

            Note: Showing resentment or hostility only gives the patient a chance to deny whatever you might imply about his underlying motives. Try again.

Answer C: *Dr.:* Since you aren't working, how are you getting along?

            Pt.: Oh, I've been getting along all right on the insurance money I collected because of this accident.

            Dr.: And this is your sole source of income?

            Pt.: Yes, there's enough to let me live easy for awhile.

            Dr.: And what will you do when that's gone?

            Pt.: Well, I hope I don't get to that point, but I might if my hand doesn't get any better, I'll have to go to work if I come to the end of what I have now.

            Note: By asking an open-ended question such as, "How are you getting along?" you have given the patient a chance to tell his own story. He has explained how he handles this situation, as well as his future plans. He has been given a chance to verbalize his feelings. (Skip to No. 4.)

Answer D: *Dr.:* How do you plan to get along if it doesn't get any better?

            Pt.: Well, I don't know—I sure can't work. (Pause.) I suppose I could apply for some kind of disability. I would certainly rather work for my board and keep, but this hand—

            Note: This is a response which gives you a good deal of information about the patient and his manifest complaint, but you have lost the key idea of the interview. Review C.

Answer E: *Dr.:* Well, just what can you do?

            Pt.: I can haul meat around just like I used to, but I have a little trouble getting it hooked up on the rack.

            Dr.: Is that all?

            Pt.: No, I just can't cut it like I used to. I just don't seem to be able to do the job as well as I once could.

Dr.: But you still can handle sides of beef pretty well?

Pt.: Yes, I'm no slouch there—just when it comes to something that you have to be careful about.

Dr.: So you can do most of your old job pretty well?

Pt.: Yes, I guess so.

Dr.: I see, and how do you plan to get along if it doesn't improve further?

> **Note:** You have asked the patient for evidence of his ability, not his disability. You have caused him to tell you what he is capable of doing. Your question has put his abilities in a positive light, along with getting further information about his work. This exchange should be very helpful since it concerns the area in which the patient is having his greatest trouble. (Continue to No. 4.)

4. *Pt.:* A lot of people have suggested that I apply for permanent disability because of my hand not improving any.

Dr.: And do you think that you could get this disability?

Pt.: I don't know.

Dr.: Is there anything else you could do?

Pt.: A friend of my wife's is a lawyer and he said that I could sue the company for loss of good use of my hand.

Dr.: And you would sue for this?

Pt.: Well, I've been thinking about it, if my hand doesn't get any better.

Dr.: Do you really feel that the company is liable for this suit?

Pt.: Look, they used to have nonskid mats on the floor for us handlers, but they took them out 2 days before I fell—said we didn't need them even on that slippery floor. I'd say they weren't considering our safety too much.

Dr.: Then you would rather sue them than go back to work?

Pt.: No, Doctor, I didn't say that, but I think I could if I wanted to.

Dr.: But you might?

Pt.: Yes, I guess I might but only if my hand gets no better.

Dr.: A. Mr. Devoe, I'm going to refer you to a friend of mine and a very good doctor who may be of more help to you. I'll give you his address and make an appointment for you (writing down the name and address of a psychiatrist).

B. Rather than sue your employer, why don't you go back to work?

C. Why don't you quit trying to buffalo me? You're able to go back to work, if you want to.

D. In view of what you have just told me, I wonder if you really want to go back to work.

Answer A: *Dr.:* Mr. Devoe, I'm going to refer you to a friend of mine and a very good doctor who may be of more help to you. I'll give you his address and make an appointment for you (writing down the name and address of a psychiatrist).

Note: You are rejecting the patient by referring him to a psychiatrist—partly to get him off your hands and partly in hope that the psychiatrist will push the right button to get the patient started again. It is unlikely that your patient will benefit at this time from psychiatric treatment because he is convinced that his problem is physical. He has not been prepared to accept a referral to a psychiatrist. All the psychiatrist can offer under this type of referral is the attachment of another diagnostic label to this uncooperative patient. To make this patient cooperative with the psychiatrist would require preparation by you, the referring doctor, so that the patient will be ready to accept emotional help. Try again.

Answer B: *Dr.:* Rather than sue your employer, why don't you go back to work?

Pt.: Because my hand is numb—you want me to get hurt again?

Dr.: You know that I don't want you hurt, but I think that you should give it a try.

Pt.: But my hand—

Dr.: I have tried to assure you that we have done about all we can for your hand at the present. I think you could work now and you tell me you couldn't possibly do so. It makes me wonder if you really want to go to work. (To response D.)

Answer C: *Dr.:* Why don't you quit trying to buffalo me? You're able to go back to work, if you want to.

Pt.: Doctor, I'm not trying to buffalo you—my hand really is numb.

Dr.: I don't care if both hands are numb. You could get out and earn your living. I've seen amputees who could do better than you are doing.

Pt.: Yes, but they got more going for them.

Dr.: And you have a whole hand going for you too. You had better try to work because I won't sign a permanent disability report for you.

Pt.: (Rising.) Okay, Doctor, but I'm sure someone else will understand my situation a lot better.

Note: You learn several months later that the patient has filed suit against the company for which he used to work. He may lose his case and opportunity for reemployment. Try again.

Answer D: *Dr.:* In view of what you have just told me, I wonder if you really want to go back to work.

Pt.: Sure, I want to, but I don't want to get hurt anymore. My hand—

Dr.: ". . . get hurt anymore?" (A reflection.)
Pt.: Yes.

> **Note:** You have challenged the patient's intentions and have asked for an explanation of his feelings. You have also used *his* words, showing understanding and at the same time signaling him to tell you more about his feelings.

Dr.: I don't understand. What are your feelings about it?
Pt.: You know how it is at work.
Dr.: No, I don't. Can you tell me about it?
Pt.: When I got hurt—my boss just didn't seem to care that I was hurt—it seems he was just sore because I was going to miss a little work.
Dr.: And did you tell him how you felt?
Pt.: Look, Doctor, I was interested in keeping my job then—I didn't want to get fired. I would have liked to have told him how I felt about his "safety program."
Dr.: And how did you feel?
Pt.: It's pretty lousy. They don't care about employee safety— they just care about how much beef they can push through that cutting room in 1 day.
Dr.: And you feel that you might get hurt again if you go back?
Pt.: A guy with one injury is a lot more likely to get another one, you know.
Dr.: How is that? (Here you challenge him.)
Pt.: (Pause.) I don't know, but it seems logical to me.
Dr.: How is that?
Pt.: It just does, I don't know why, but isn't that right?
Dr.: One can't really be sure, but at this point it seems to be a feeling you have and not necessarily a fact.
Pt.: (Pause.) Now that you put it that way, I guess you are right, but I still feel that I'm right.
Dr.: Let's review the time before when you went back to work for a few days—did you have an accident then?
Pt.: No, guess I didn't.
Dr.: But you thought you might?
Pt.: Well, you see—I was being extra careful since I had only been out of the hospital a week.
Dr.: Then you mean you weren't yourself. You weren't at ease with the job.
Pt.: Yes, you remember the rubber mat they took out before my accident?
Dr.: (Nods.)
Pt.: It still hasn't been put back.
Dr.: Would you agree, then, that you are more concerned about your safety. It has become an important focus for you.
Pt.: How do you figure that?
Dr.: Use your few days at work as an example.

Pt.: (Thinks a minute.) Yes, you are right, Doctor. Maybe my concern is out of proportion but it still makes me uneasy.

Note: You have, by your series of responses, made the patient conscious of his previously unconscious fears. You have made it possible for him to admit to you his fears without embarrassment. After telling you of his feelings about work he can view his own attitude objectively rather than emotionally. He had previously reacted only to intrinsic emotions or to feelings he has had about his employment. He may now react with more logic by bringing the problem into consciousness. By helping the patient to realize and accept (as well as to deal with) his feelings, you have helped him mature. With this more mature attitude he may very well be more motivated to return to work.

MR. NEWTON: a defensive patient

Mr. Newton, a 25-year-old married, white male, comes into your office. You are at your desk (rise, shake hands, note a limp, flabby handshake) and you ask him to be seated.

1. *Dr.:* Good morning, Mr. Newton. What's the trouble?

    Pt.: Suppose you tell me, Doc—that's what I'm here to find out.

Follow the instructions given at the beginning of the interview with Mr. Devoe (p. 112).

    Dr.: A. How do you expect me to help you with an attitude like that? If you don't tell me all you can, I can't hope to be of any assistance to you.

           B. Well, let's not be too unreasonable, after all I need some information to work with. I am certain we can find out with your cooperation. Now what is the trouble?

           C. I'm here to help you if you'll only cooperate with me. Now, just calm down and let's talk reasonably about this.

           D. I am not a veterinarian. There is one across the street if that is what you want.

           E. There must be something troubling you.

Answer A: *Dr.* How do you expect me to help you with an attitude like that? If you don't tell me all you can, I can't hope to be of any assistance to you.

        Note: Replying with obvious frustration, as you just have, is what the patient expects of you. His original statement is an indication of how he wants you to feel to justify his anger. His likely response to your obvious frustration is, "You see, what did I tell you, you're mad already because I didn't say what you expected me to." Select another response.

Answer B: *Dr.* Well, let's not be too unreasonable, after all I need some information to work with. I am certain we can find out with your cooperation. Now what is the trouble?

Pt.: What do you mean you need other information to work with? You asked me again what the trouble was—that's why I came to see you. I don't *know*. Do you expect me to diagnose my own case? (See answer C.)

Answer C: *Dr.:* I'm here to help you if you'll only cooperate with me. Now just calm down and let's talk reasonably about this.

> **Note:** You have just managed to lose your professional edge by being defensive in response to the patient. After all, Doctor, it's not your fault the patient is angry. He was angry before he came in. You fell for his bait. Select another response.

Answer D: *Dr.:* I am not a veterinarian. There is one across the street if that is what you want.

> **Note:** There are two possible alternatives to this:
> (1) The patient says, "Well, Doctor, if you're going to sit and insult me to my face, I can go elsewhere." This is a situation where the patient becomes outraged at being "insulted" by the gruff or blunt manner in which you reacted. This response will only be tolerated by those patients who have a positive rapport with the doctor.
> (2) The patient says, "Okay, Doc, I guess you're right—I was being foolish."
> *Dr.:* That's all right, Mr. Newton, now what did you come to see me about?
> *Pt.:* Well, there's this pain I have been having in my stomach.
> This is the situation where the patient realized his actions were inappropriate. You have sidestepped the barrier of anger and can go on with the interview. (Skip to No. 2.)

Answer E: *Dr.:* There must be something troubling you.
Pt.: Yes, there is something bothering me, Doctor, and I guess I haven't been much help to you. The trouble I have is—well, my stomach has been bothering me lately.

> **Note:** You have successfully penetrated the anger reaction to reach the latent content or source of anger and you may get on with the interview. (Skip to No. 2.)

2. *Dr.:* A pain in your stomach—can you tell me more about it?
Pt.: I noticed it first when I ate some cabbage. It stays about here (indicates region of pylorus).

Dr.:   A.   Could you define this pain?
           B.   What's it like?
           C.   How long does it last?
           D.   Is it sharp?

Answer A: *Dr.:*   Could you define this pain?

                Pt.:   Yes, it sort of just stays right about where I showed you. It's a pretty dull pain. It doesn't double me over or anything.

                Note: This is fairly specific information for the patient to relate at this time. It would be advisable to seek more diverse information to obtain a more accurate picture of how the illness happened—when, where, and with whom (under what circumstances). Select another response.

Answer B: *Dr.:*   What's it like?

                Pt.:   Well, it's a dull pain—it keeps me from lying in bed too long.

                Dr.:   Oh, how's that?

                Pt.:   Well—I find if I eat some breakfast, it goes away. It generally isn't too bad after meals, or if I drink some milk at work.

                Dr.:   When did you first notice this?

                Pt.:   Oh, about a month ago, no (pause) let's see (pause) Fred died 5 weeks ago and it started about a week and a half later—about 3½ weeks ago, doctor.

                Note: You have asked for the general picture and have received a good deal of information. You have received quite a bit more than you would have obtained through the same number of responses by asking specific questions about limited aspects of the patient's condition. (Skip to No. 3.)

Answer C: *Dr.:*   How long does it last?

                Pt.:   Oh, not too long.

                Dr.:   Does it burn?

                Pt.:   Yes, sometimes it does.

                Dr.:   Where, exactly, does it hurt you?

                Pt.:   Oh, right about here, where I showed you before (again indicates region of abdomen at about the pylorus). It's pretty hard to pin down exactly.

                Dr.:   You said it doesn't last too long—could you be more specific?

                Pt.:   Oh, I don't know, 30 or 40 minutes maybe.

                Note: See answer A for explanation of this sequence.

Answer D: *Dr.:*   Is it sharp?

Pt.: A little sharp.

Dr.: Does it come and go?

Pt.: Yes, I suppose it does.

Dr.: Does milk help it?

Pt.: Yes, sometimes when I drink some milk it will ease up a little.

> **Note:** You are leading the patient toward his response. You are asking direct yes-no questions that will elicit mostly *yes* answers. The fact that the patient first experienced trouble after eating some cabbage does not necessarily prove that he has gallbladder trouble, although this is a frequent symptom. You are not allowing the patient freedom or respecting his opinions. You are working for a predetermined diagnosis, not for an understanding of the patient. The two are not always synonymous. Select another response.

3. **Comment:** You have been questioning the patient about the onset of his symptoms. He has replied, "Oh, about a month ago (pause) let's see, Fred died 5 weeks ago, and it started about a week and a half later—about 3½ weeks ago." What is your reply to this?

Dr.: A. He died?
B. Has your pain changed during this 3½-week interval?
C. What were you doing at that time?
D. Was it a dull pain then?

Answer A: *Dr.:* He died?

Pt.: Yes, it was all real sudden. He had a heart attack right on the job—Oh, I'm sorry, Doc, I didn't tell you, Fred was my boss.

Dr.: I see—this must have been pretty upsetting.

Pt.: I guess it was for a while. He was there one minute, and (gestures) poof! gone the next.

> **Note:** You have correctly surmised an emotional reaction of the patient to the death of his employer. Go on with the program and determine his involvement and relationship with his new employer. (Skip to No. 4.)

Answer B: *Dr.:* Has your pain changed during this 3½-week interval?

Pt.: No, it's always about the same.

Dr.: Always the same?

Pt.: Yes, it really doesn't change too much at all. It has been getting a little worse lately.

> **Note:** You are diligently getting the chronologic progress of the symptoms, but overlooking some pertinent facts mentioned by the patient. Try again.

Answer C: *Dr.:* What were you doing at that time?
Pt.: Oh, working—same as usual.

> **Note:** You are diligently getting the chronologic progress of the symptoms, but overlooking some pertinent facts mentioned by the patient. Try again.

Answer D: *Dr.:* Was it a dull pain then?
Pt.: Yes, about the same, only not as frequent.
Dr.: Was it in about the same spot?
Pt.: That's right—it hasn't moved around any.
Dr.: Then this hasn't changed a lot?
Pt.: No, except it's more frequent now.

> **Note:** The information obtained by this series of questions is very specific and concentrates on details before a general understanding is obtained. These questions also miss important information. Try again.

4. *Dr.:* How did you feel about this?
Pt.: Well, I guess I was pretty upset. I'll never have another boss like Fred.
Dr.: He treated you pretty well? (*or,* You were pretty close friends?)
Pt.: Yes, Fred would respect you for what you were, not like some of these other slave drivers that see you as a piece of machinery, instead of the person you are.
Dr.: How do you feel about work now?
Pt.: Oh, Mr. K. is all right, but nothing like Fred. He doesn't seem to see that you can't do everything. He expects you to be a superman around the shop.
Dr.: He doesn't respect you then?
Pt.: No, not really.
Dr.: How has today been?
Pt.: Well, I got up feeling as I usually do, ate breakfast, and went to work at 8:00. I punched in and went into Mr. K.'s office to tell him I had this appointment with you at 1:00. He just looked up from behind his desk, frowned at me, and said, "Okay, just get back as soon as possible," as if he were going to lose 10 or 15 minutes of production while I was gone. My stomach starting hurting about 9:30, so I drank a carton of milk and it quieted down. It acts like it's going to start up again.
Dr.: Oh, what do you notice?
Pt.: Well, there's this burning feeling, like indigestion, and I feel a little sick. I really notice it at night. I sleep pretty well, usually. Have a little trouble getting to sleep sometimes.
Dr.: What seems to keep you awake?
Pt.: I guess I worry a little too much.
Dr.: About?
Pt.: Oh, whether or not I'll keep this job with Mr. K. there. My wife says I'm foolish to worry about it, but I don't know.

Dr.: A. You should be pretty secure in your job, I would think. After all, you have been working there some time.

B. How's that?

C. I wouldn't worry if I were you—you'll be all right—you're a good worker.

Answer A: *Dr.:* You should be pretty secure in your job, I would think. After all, you have been working there some time.

Pt.: Maybe I should be, but I'm not.

Dr.: Well, why aren't you?

Pt.: That's what I have been trying to tell you.

Note: You are not telling the patient anything he isn't already aware of. You are merely adding to his anxiety by failing to understand his feeling. He feels he should not be worried, but still he is and doesn't fully understand his worry. Why don't you encourage the patient to tell you more? It is to your advantage to have him talk out his feeling. Talking usually leads to further understanding by both the patient and the physician. Try again.

Answer B: *Dr.:* How's that?

Pt.: Oh, I just don't know if Mr. K. will keep me or not.

Dr.: Would he have any reason for not employing you?

Pt.: Not that I know of, but the little things really bother him.

Dr.: Little things?

Pt.: Yes, like taking a few more minutes for a coffee break than we're supposed to, that sort of thing.

Dr.: And he gets on your back about this?

Pt.: Yes, I spend about half my day looking at my watch—I really can't stand this guy.

Note: By allowing the patient a good deal of freedom in answering, and by showing your concern, you have encouraged the patient to reveal his feelings about his job and employer. He is, in fact, telling you what bothers him. (Skip to No. 5.)

Answer C: *Dr.:* I wouldn't worry if I were you—you'll be all right—you're a good worker.

Pt.: You wouldn't worry about it?

Dr.: No, I think not.

Pt.: Not even with this guy breathing down your neck every minute?

Dr.: You still do a pretty good job, don't you?

Pt.: Yes, I guess so—am I crazy or something to feel this way?

Note: How can you tell the patient how he should feel? Feelings are very private information. Are you telling him you could do a better job of controlling your feelings in his situation? About what are you trying to reassure him? Do you feel you have to negate his feeling of unworthiness by denying it, or making it seem illogical? See this problem from the patient's viewpoint. Save your suggestions until you have the whole story. Try again.

5. Comment: The patient has just related that he spends "about half my day looking at my watch—I really can't stand this guy." The patient has stated both his dislike for his employer, and the anxiety he feels for the day to end. Which of the following responses will you choose in response to his statement?

    Dr.: A. Have you felt this way about other employers?
             B. You don't like Mr. K., do you?
             C. Were you afraid you might be late for this appointment?

Answer A: *Dr.:* Have you felt this way about other employers?
          Pt.: Well, yes, I suppose I have. They all expect you to work like a slave and to be treated like a dog.
          Dr.: All of them?
          Pt.: Well, all but Fred.
          Dr.: And Mr. K. is like the rest of them?
          Pt.: Yes, a lot like the rest.
          Dr.: And they expect a lot from you?
          Pt.: Yes, they're pretty unreasonable.
          Dr.: In what way?
          Pt.: Oh, they jump on you for a lot of little things, you know, *little* things.

          Note: You have been exploring the patient's feelings about his past experiences. The feelings he has had previously will be likely to carry on into the present. This information will help you to understand the patient. Now go to response C.

Answer B: *Dr.:* You don't like Mr. K., do you?
          Pt.: No—but he's all right, I guess—he's a pretty good boss, as bosses go.

          Note: You're being a little bit too specific. Mr. K. is probably just a symbol for something else. Try again.

Answer C: *Dr.:* Were you afraid you might be late for this appointment?
          Pt.: Well, I didn't want to come in late. I didn't want to run you behind schedule.
          Dr.: Were you afraid I might give you a hard time if you were late?
          Pt.: You wouldn't have been too happy about it, would you?
          Dr.: I think I could have worked around it, without too much trouble—but at any rate, I wouldn't have scolded you.

Pt.: Well, I guess I am just used to catching it for being late. I was afraid you might complain about it too.

Dr.: And this upsets you?

Pt.: Well, sure it does. I am tired of these straw bosses chewing me out for little things like that.

Note: If you chose this response to follow—"Were you afraid you might be late for this appointment," you have jumped the gun. It might be best to work through a history of the patient's past experiences and to develop some empathy for the patient's feelings in this secton, before exploring present events. Try again if you have chosen answer C.

If you chose answer A, you will notice that here you have uncovered the reason for the initial hostility you encountered when the patient came in to see you. He was afraid you would scold him for being a minute late.

Comment: You may now proceed with questions about specific symptoms of the patient's physical condition. You may want to get diagnostic roentgenograms of the patient's abdomen. Whatever your further course, the patient's tension has been made apparent by this interview allowing the patient to deal with it. You can more clearly realize why the patient was hostile when he came in to see you. You are a very definite authority figure to him, and he has much difficulty in relating to authority figures. Therefore, as an authority figure, you received much of the patient's accumulated hostility toward these people. You can see the necessity for him to release this emotion before you can conduct a successful interview.

MRS. BROWN: a testing patient

Mrs. Brown is a 40-year-old, married, white female. This is her first visit. The nurse reports the chief complaint as "stomach pains." As Mrs. Brown enters, she says, "Good morning, Doctor. I'm Mrs. Brown. Eileen G. told me you might be able to help me."

Dr.: What seems to be the trouble?

Pt.: I've been having these pains in my stomach.

Dr.: Pains in your stomach?

Pt.: They have been giving me an awful lot of trouble and I'm about crazy with them.

Dr.: Can you tell me more about them?

Pt.: Well, the pains start right about here (indicates lower sternal area) and sometimes down here as well (indicates right flank). It's sort of a burning feeling and at times it cramps.

Dr.: When do you notice these pains?

Pt.: Oh, just every so often, like early in the morning, when I bend over to get the clothes out of the washer and almost anytime, day or night. Are you married Doctor?

Follow the instructions given at the beginning of the interview with Mr. Devoe (p. 112).

Dr.: A. Yes, I am.

        B. Why do you ask?

Answer A: *Dr.:* Yes, I am.

            Pt.: But you look so young to be married.

            Dr.: No younger than my wife looks (he smiles).

            Pt.: I've always—is it possible for one to be married to a Doctor and still have a happy home?

            Dr.: Well, we think so—now about your stomach pains.

            Pt.: (Interrupting.) Just one more thing Doctor—does your wife think she is lucky to have you?

                Note: You have given the patient a chance to corner you and take control of this interview. This sequence of responses on your part encourages the patient to persist in her mode of response. If you have not read answer B, do so. If you have, skip to No. 1.

Answer B: *Dr.:* Why do you ask?
Pt.: I was just curious.
Dr.: I see, can you tell me why?

> **Note:** Here you query the patient about her question and challenge the patient's question of your marital status. This lets her know that such questions are not a part of the role of patient. This is necessary to break into her mode of responses. Review answer A to see the dilemma you could have gotten into by simply answering her question.

1. *Dr.:* I see, can you tell me why?
Pt.: Well, then you know how your wife works around the house, what she has to do—how she has to work there by herself.
Dr.: Being home must bother you!
Pt.: Yes, it's not a pleasant life. You seem to already know how I suffer. You certainly are considerate.
Dr.: A. Now, Mrs. Brown, I assure you I try to be considerate with all my patients. Now how long have you had these pains?
    B. Tell me more about these pains.
    C. Mrs. Brown, I really can't say that I know how you suffer yet, I don't have enough information. How long have you had these pains?

Answer A: *Dr.:* Now, Mrs. Brown, I assure you I try to be considerate with all my patients. Now how long have you had these pains?

> **Note:** You are denying the patient the feeling she wants to have of exclusive care. Is it frightening that she profusely compliments you? You are telling her that you do not see her any differently than the rest of your patients. You then scold her effectively by saying, "Come on now, let's get along with this, quit dragging your feet." She has a reason to compliment you. Look at the patient's need and the ways she is testing you. Try again.

Answer B: *Dr.:* Tell me more about these pains.
Pt.: What do you mean?
Dr.: Oh, how long have you had them. Have they changed? What have you noticed about them?

> **Note:** In an attempt to avoid hard work, guessing, and an unproductive question-answer session, you deliberately ask more than one question at a time to encourage the patient to talk more freely.

Pt.: Oh, I just noticed a sharp pain in my stomach while fixing breakfast 3 weeks ago. I believe it was Sunday morning, oh, yes, it was, because I remember going in and waking Harvey because it was so severe.

Dr.: And then.

Pt.: He was no help, all he could say was, "Mama, why do you bother me this early after being out late last night?" So then I ate some cereal and got some relief.

Dr.: The cereal seemed to relieve the pain?

Pt.: Yes, it did very quickly.

Dr.: Does anything else seem to help? (Skip to No. 2.)

Answer C: *Dr.:* Mrs. Brown, I really can't say that I know how you suffer yet, I don't have enough information. How long have you had these pains?

Pt.: I would think you should know how I suffer—you're such a good Doctor.

Dr.: I still need some more information from you before I can begin to—

Pt.: (Interrupts.) Oh, you can just look at me and tell what's wrong, can't you? You are just being modest, Doctor, you know what's wrong but you just don't want to worry me.

Dr.: That's not entirely true.

Note: See answer A and try again.

2. *Pt.:* Thank goodness, I have Alka-Seltzer. I take two or three of them and sit down awhile and the pain goes away. You look tired, Doctor, you must certainly work long hours.

Dr.: A. Let's confine ourselves to your stomach trouble at the present— you say you sit down awhile and the pain goes away, does anything else help?

B. You would work long hours, too, if you had the overhead I have, now, what else seems to help this pain?

C. Perhaps I do, what else seems to help the pain?

D. You seem to have something important you would like to tell me?

Answer A: *Dr.:* Let's confine ourselves to your stomach trouble at the present. You say you sit down awhile and the pain goes away, does anything else help?

Pt.: No, that's about all, I guess.

Dr.: And have you had them long?

Pt.: No, only a few days—they will pass, I suppose.

Dr.: Have you ever noticed them previous to the past 3 weeks?

Pt.: No, this is the first time I have ever noticed them.

Dr.: And does your husband ever notice it?

Pt.: No, he just sits there and never notices anything.

Dr.: What else can you tell me about the pains?

Pt.: There's not much to tell, Doctor. If you will just give me something to keep the pain down, I'll stop taking up your time. I know you must be busy.

Note: You have denied the patient her method of building you up, without getting to the possible cause for it. She is mentally creating a wonderful person in you for some reason. Because of her persistence, perhaps you should find out why. Since she has lost the possibility of building you up, she has denied much of her illness. She has given up because you refuse to let her gain confidence by relating to you in an overcomplimentary way. Try again.

Answer B: *Dr.:* You would work long hours, too, if you had the overhead I have, now, what else seems to help this pain?

Pt.: Nothing much.

Note: You have given the patient the impression that your long hours are not a result of the interest in your patients—ergo this patient—but rather a result of interest in your financial condition. Contrary to what you told the medical school admission committee, you really hate people and love money. Try again.

Answer C: *Dr.:* Perhaps I do, what else seems to help the pain?

Pt.: Oh, not much of anything—Harvey just sits around and grumbles when I complain. He's a good man, but he doesn't listen much. I'll bet you don't ignore your wife, doctor!

Note: You have sidestepped the patient's response one more time; but you have run into the same mode of response from the patient. You have done nothing to ascertain the patient's reason for these profuse compliments. To continue with the patient's history, it will be necessary to eliminate this type of response by uncovering the reason for her compliments. Try again.

Answer D: *Dr.:* You seem to have something important you would like to tell me?

Pt.: Well, (hesitates) yes and no, doctor.

Dr.: Can you explain what you mean by that?

Pt.: I would like to tell you, but I am not sure you would understand.

Dr.: I will try to understand if you can tell me about it.

Pt.: My Harvey—well, an understanding person he isn't. So I'll tell you Doctor, I pray you will understand and won't throw me out.

Note: You have correctly acted on the assumption that the patient has been complimenting you because she wanted to tell you something that is very difficult for her to talk about. Now, find out what it is. (Go to No. 3.)

3. *Dr.:* What's the situation?
   Pt.: My son, Sheldon—you know my son. He's married now—ran out of his own home to be with this girl. If I told him once, I told him a hundred times—"Sheldon," I said, "you've got to watch or you will be a papa already. So now a papa he is going to be."
   Dr.: And when did you learn this?
   Pt.: Oh, about a month ago, he comes in and says "Mama—I have good news—I am going to be married to a wonderful girl." I say—"So, you want a medal? Lots of people get married—happens every day." Then he tells me it's a week from then and the wedding is set and am I happy. I say, sure we are happy. I call Harvey and then go up to my room and break down. It's not every day you lose your only son, who is 23 years old and never been away from home, a son who doesn't even know how to handle his money good yet.
   Dr.: And what did you do then?
   Pt.: So what else could I do? The next day I told Sheldon I was ashamed of crying and that it was wonderful he was going to be married. The next Sunday we went to the wedding and I managed to last through it. I have never cried so hard, Doctor, as when Sheldon and that girl left us at the church.
   Dr.: It was hard to see him leave!
   Pt.: It sure was. He meant a lot to me.
   Dr.: And since then?
   Pt.: Like a good mother, I have wished him and his wife well, but it's awfully lonely at home with Harvey—who, bless his heart, doesn't say, "How are you Mama?" or "How's the weather?"—just sits there, reading his newspaper and eating the food I fix him.
   Dr.: What can you do about the loneliness?
   Pt.: Oh,—that's the hard part. You'll think an old woman like me is crazy, Doctor, but I do all I can and—(Pause.)
   Dr.: And then?
   Pt.: I drink a little Doctor. When Harvey gets in bed in the evening, I sit up, and I tell him it's the late show I'm watching, but that's when, heaven forbid, I pour myself a drink.

   Dr.: A. And how long have you been doing this?
         B. Do you drink a great deal like this?
         C. Don't you know that's not the way to solve your problem?
         D. And then?

Answer A: *Dr.:* And how long have you been doing this?
             Pt.: Oh, for the past few weeks.
             Dr.: Is this the only time you drink?
             Pt.: Well, no, I have a few drinks in the morning after Harvey leaves, so I won't feel bad.
             Dr.: What do you mean by a few drinks?
             Pt.: Just a few.

             Note: You have accepted the situation, as the patient

has been building you up to do. You have listened to the confession without judging or scolding her, but without supporting her either. You have proceeded as a machine would proceed. You must also show that you are human as well. Show a little more concern and feeling. After all the patient is concerned about it. She seems to have strong feelings about it, so show that you realize this. Here you are being too distant. A little empathy goes a long way. Try again.

Answer B: *Dr.:* Do you drink a great deal like this?
Pt.: No, not a lot.

> **Note:** You should emphasize positive aspects to your patient, not possible negative ones. "Great deal" of drinking might possibly connote alcoholism to her. A better question here might be, "About how many drinks do you have every evening?" Even this type of question is somewhat impersonal and cold. Try again.

Answer C: *Dr.:* Don't you know that's not the way to solve your problem?
Pt.: I know it isn't the way to solve my problem. But I thought you would understand.
Dr.: I understand your loneliness and the feeling you have that you need a drink, but you must realize it is not the best thing to do.

> **Note:** How do you know it is not the best of alternatives in her specific situation? It may well be better than taking some medication, or taking her life.

Pt.: Don't you think I realize that? Why do you think I came to you?

> **Note:** You are telling the patient something of which she was already aware and ashamed. She felt that she had to build you up so that you would accept her complaint without adding to her guilt. You may feel strongly about solitary drinking, but you must understand as well the patient's need to talk about it freely. You are giving advice as if you could live better in her situation than she does. What right do you have to tell her what she should or should not do? Try again.

Answer D: *Dr.:* And then?
Pt.: Then I feel a little better, so I generally just pour another couple of drinks.
Dr.: Does this seem to relax you?
Pt.: Not really—but I can go to sleep. Oh, poor Harvey, if he knew what his miserable wife does.

Dr.: This must be very disturbing to you! (Empathic response.)

Pt.: Oh, yes, it's a terrible strain, just terrible—but what else can I do? I'm afraid he may find the empty bottles. When he leaves for work, I have a few more drinks.

Dr.: I see—about how much do you drink?

> **Note:** You have accepted the patient's feelings; you have shown her respect and have shown that you will try to understand her problem. She has spoken freely of her situation at home, one which she feels strongly about. This is the situation for which she had been building you up previously by complimenting you. She must feel that you are a wonderful doctor and a warm, understanding person before she can relate her problems to you. This reply "and then?" was not distant, but it implied to the patient that you wanted her to continue the story in her fashion, that her comments interested you, and that you respected her ability to tell the story. (To No. 4.)

4. *Pt.:* Oh, two or three, about the same as I have at night.

Dr.: And do you get up with these pains?

Pt.: Yes, I do.

Dr.: And when does it seem to get better?

Pt.: Well, I take these morning drinks so I won't feel too low. It gets better especially after breakfast, and it seems to improve. I have a big breakfast with cereal instead of just toast and coffee.

Dr.: You mentioned that you first noticed the pain after being out late on Saturday night—what did you do the night before?

Pt.: We were at the annual bowling party. Everyone was drinking and having a good time. I remember I had more than I usually do.

Dr.: And how much do you usually drink at a party?

Pt.: Oh, not enough to make me tipsy, just enough so I can relax and enjoy the party.

Dr.: Does this make you feel relaxed?

Pt.: Yes, I feel pretty relaxed after three or four drinks.

Dr.: Lately, you have about this same amount in the evenings as in the mornings?

Pt.: Yes, every day for the past 2 weeks or so.

Dr.: How would your husband feel if he knew you were doing this?

Pt.: Heaven preserve me, he might disown me—his own wife—if he knew.

Dr.: And how does this make you feel?

Pt.: (Pause, hesitantly)—ashamed that he will feel like throwing me out for this foolishness.

Dr.: Ashamed?

Pt.: Yes, I suppose I feel ashamed because of my bad habits and afraid of what this will lead to.

Dr.: Like what?

Pt.: My older brother was an alcoholic. He died from liver disease. I knew what he went through, as they lived up the street and I saw him daily.

Dr.: That must be pretty frightening to think about.

Comment: You have shown empathy and are ready to have the patient define alternative behavior that you can support. From a further interview with the patient, you will be able to discover possible alternatives available to her in overcoming her loneliness and in avoiding the drinking. You may also enlist the assistance of a public health nurse, minister, marriage counselor, social worker, or social organization to help this desperate patient through this difficult situation. With the additional information you have just derived, her history of pain follows that which you might expect to be associated with episodes of alcoholic gastritis. With the patient's drinking habits in mind, this is quite likely a reasonable assumption. Further physical and laboratory examination and follow-up of a comprehensive (medical-psychiatric) treatment program should confirm your diagnosis and reverse the progression of this illness.

INTERVIEW 6

MRS. MONROE: a manipulative patient

Mrs. Monroe is an elderly widow whom you have known for a number of years. She is the family matriarch. She dominates her children. She gives them extensive financial aid and expensive gifts. In return she demands much catering and attention. She has marked cardiac disease and uses this as a crutch to strengthen her position with them in times of stress. She comes into your office complaining of a pain in her chest. After examining her you find no new abnormalities in comparison to previous visits. Your reply is an attempt to relieve some of the problems of the patient and her family.

Follow the instructions given at the beginning of the interview with Mr. Devoe (p. 112).

1. *Dr.:* A. Mrs. Monroe, after going over you, I find no change in your heart condition. I am going to prescribe something that will help you relax, but I want you to know you have nothing to cause you any added concern.
   B. Now, Mrs. Monroe, I don't believe you have a reasonable excuse for coming in today. I think you are causing yourself and your family a lot of unnecessary worry and expense by putting so much emphasis on your heart condition when it doesn't appear to have changed since your last visit.
   C. The examination indicates no change in your heart condition since your last visit. How are things going along at home?

Answer A: *Dr.:* Mrs. Monroe, after going over you, I find no change in your heart condition. I am going to prescribe something that will help you relax, but I want you to know you have nothing to cause you any added concern.
   Pt.: You mean there's nothing I should worry about?
   Dr.: That is my opinion.
   Pt.: And you think I should go home and stop worrying?
   Dr.: As long as you continue your medication, I see no reason you should feel concerned.
   Pt.: I feel better already.

Note: The patient returns to her family feeling serene in her old role. You have just reinforced this role by giving it professional sanction. She will return to you time after time with the same complaint. Nothing has been altered. She controls her family partly with her symptoms. Rather than improving the patient's condition, you have reinforced it and have added unnecessarily to the expense of her medical care. Reread the statement and try again.

Answer B: *Dr.:* Now, Mrs. Monroe, I don't believe you have a reasonable excuse for coming in today. I think you are causing yourself and your family a lot of unnecessary worry and expense by putting so much emphasis on your heart condition when it doesn't appear to have changed since your last visit.

Pt.: Well, Doctor, I know there is something wrong, and I'd call a heart condition a reason to see you. If you're going to talk that way to me, I'll take my condition to someone who is more concerned with his patients.

Note: You have antagonized her with response B. There is a strong possibility the patient actually will go to a different physician. This will put both the physician and the patient at a disadvantage. The possibility of her coming back hinges upon your professional relationship with her and her confidence in you. (Skip to No. 2.)

Answer C: *Dr.:* The examination indicates no change in your heart condition since your last visit. How are things going along at home?

Pt.: Suzi has been with her children for the past 2 weeks, and John is away on his new job.

Dr.: You have been all alone.

Note: You might want to say: "How do you feel about this," or something quite similar. This is the place to show empathy, and recognition of the patient's feelings by letting her know that you do recognize them. You don't have to do any high-powered deduction to sense the patient's feelings.

Pt.: Yes, the four walls and the cat get pretty dull.

Dr.: You have no one to talk to then.

Pt.: Well, my neighbor was a real pal to me—we talked a lot, but she died last month.

Dr.: How has this affected you?

Pt.: I just don't have anyone to talk to anymore. I can't get through the days without feeling lonely. There's nothing much I can do about it unless the children are home.

Dr.: What do you do when the children are with you?

Pt.: Oh, we sit around and talk, and I play with the grand-children. It's so good to have them with me.

Dr.: So you now rely more upon your children for your companionship?

Pt.: Yes, Doctor—they're about all I have—I know I depend on them far too much. I just don't feel that I have much of anything when I'm all by myself.

Dr.: How do your children feel about this?

Pt.: I really don't know, Doctor—I can't seem to keep them around me much. I suppose any mother would want her children closer to her.

Dr.: And how do you keep them close to you?

Pt.: I just try to be as nice to them as I can. Oh, we have fallings-out sometimes, but we always make up.

Dr.: How do you go about making up?

Pt.: I usually give the children something to make up for the trouble I have caused them.

Dr.: You give your children gifts?

Pt.: Yes—like Suzi and I had a disagreement about the baby's christening. Later, after we had both cooled off, I gave her the money for the baby's christening clothes.

Dr.: Why do you suppose you do this?

Pt.: I don't know—I suppose I have done it ever since they were children.

Note: You are on the right track, you have moved to examples of Mrs. Monroe's problems with her family. Using this type of interview you may go on to allow her to release her feelings. It may take several sessions with you, using an interview of this sort, to effectively resolve the problems. You have seen how the latent content of an interview can complicate a patient's condition and treatment. In this case, the frustration Mrs. Monroe is undergoing has not yet complicated her heart condition. But you cannot ignore this distinct possibility should she continue to suffer the same frustrations. If you did not select response B, go back and do so, the results may interest you.

2. The patient leaves, angry. You discover later that she has gone back to her four walls and her cat, and has been sick in bed at her home, for the past 3 days, with at least one of her children there at all times. A few days after you learn this, however, you are given the blessing of another of her visits. She is escorted in by your office nurse and is carrying a small package.

Dr.: Good afternoon, Mrs. Monroe. What brings you here today?

Pt.: I want you to write another prescription for my heart pills. I seem to have lost the original, and I'm out of them.

Dr.: Well, that can be arranged (gets out prescription pad).

Pt.: I'm ashamed of the way I acted on my last visit to you. I think I should apologize for my behavior. (She places the small package on the desk.) Here, Doctor, this is for you and your wife. I thought you might enjoy it.

Dr.: Now, Mrs. Monroe, you know that's not necessary.

Pt.: Yes, Doctor, I know I have caused you a great deal of trouble and I want to make up for it.

Dr.: A. Seeing that she will be disappointed if you do not accept her gift, you respond, "All right, if it will make you happy, but I don't feel that I have earned it."

B. Realizing the meaning behind her actions you reply, "No, Mrs. Monroe, I'm afraid I cannot accept your gift. Professional ethics ask that we receive nothing from patients except that which we bill for services. I appreciate your gesture, but I cannot accept your gift."

C. "Thank you, Mrs. Monroe" (leaving gift on desk, unopened). "I appreciate your consideration, but I wonder if you feel there is something about your last visit that makes this gift necessary?"

Answer A: *Dr.: Seeing that she will be disappointed if you do not accept her gift, you respond:* All right, if it will make you happy, but I don't feel that I have earned it.

Pt.: Oh, I believe you have, Doctor.

Note: She is right, Doctor, but you haven't earned your fee. You have just behaved the way she expects her children to act, and you have earned the same position she has created for them. You have also violated your code of ethics, for when you open the wrapped gift there lies a $100 bill. This is not a reasonable gift is it? She has always bought friendship and now she has bought yours as well. You have perpetuated her neurotic method of trying to buy friendship and trying to undo her own hostile acts. Try again.

Answer B: *Dr.: Realizing the meaning behind her actions you reply:* No, Mrs. Monroe, I'm afraid I cannot accept your gift. Professional ethics ask that we receive nothing from patients except that which we bill for services. I appreciate your gesture, but I cannot accept your gift.

Note: You have practiced ethically, but you haven't practiced comprehensive medicine. She still doesn't understand why she thought it was a good idea to give you the gift or why she is attempting to treat you as she does her children. You have ignored the latent content of her act. You have not helped her or altered her behavior. Try again.

Answer C: *Dr.:* Thank you, Mrs. Monroe (leaving gift on desk, unopened). I appreciate your consideration, but I wonder if you feel there is something about your last visit that makes this gift necessary?

Pt.: Because I thought it was the right thing to do.

Dr.: Oh, how come? (Confrontation.)

Pt.: Well, you were mad at me, weren't you? When I thought about it at home alone, it seemed that you were very angry with me..

Dr.: Is that how it seemed to you?

Pt.: Well, you said that I wasn't really sick, and implied that I was taking up your time, and too much of the children's time, with my heart condition.

Dr.: Do you always give gifts to those who you feel are mad at you?

Pt.: Not always but it helps heal things, I think.

Dr.: Do you give them to your children?

Pt.: Yes, I do, but we don't have many arguments.

Dr.: You have done this for some time? (It is obvious that such behavior has gone on for a long time. Thus, your statement shows your understanding and leads the patient to discuss the origin of the behavior.)

Pt.: Yes, I suppose so—ever since they were little children.

Dr.: And has it always helped "heal things" for you?

Pt.: Well, I don't believe it has hurt anything.

Dr.: Do you feel this is necessary?

Pt.: Not really—but it's all I have, Doctor. (She begins to cry.) I'm just a lonely old mother and not very important any more (continues to cry).

Dr.: A. Here now, stop crying and we'll talk about what's bothering you (soothing tone).

   B. (Silence.)

   C. What are you thinking?

   D. (Patting her shoulder.) Now Mrs. Monroe—I'm sure it is uncomfortable to talk about this, but can you tell me more?

   E. How do you mean unimportant? What do you mean when you say it is all you have? (You challenge the patient.)

Answer A: *Dr.:* Here now, stop crying, and we'll talk about what's bothering you (soothing tone).

   Note: What does her crying mean to you that you cannot let her cry? It is to your advantage to let her cry. She needs to be able to cry in front of you and to be able to talk about this disturbing situation of being an old, unwanted mother. Do not be afraid to let her cry for it is usually a way of asking for help. Try again.

Answers B and C: (The patient stops crying.)

Dr.: Tell me what thoughts you have just had.

Pt.: It all seems so useless.

Dr.: In what way?

Pt.: Everything I try to do is criticized and doesn't seem to help. (Skip to No. 3.)

Answer D: *Dr.:* (Patting her shoulder.) Now Mrs. Monroe—I'm sure it is uncomfortable to talk about this, but can you tell me more?

> **Note:** Tears are a remarkably seductive agent. With an elderly widow of Mrs. Monroe's age, it is probably safe to pat her on the shoulder, but don't count yourself safe in all such cases. Furthermore, the tears are to your advantage. You did not hurt her feelings, so stop being defensive. Crying before you may be a way of testing you to see how much you can accept and understand from a patient. If you can accept the patient's tears and continue the line of thought, you will score high on this test. Crying may also be a way of avoiding a topic. In this case her defense of blocking further questioning will fail if you continue the topic. Try again.

Answer E: *Dr.:* How do you mean unimportant? What do you mean it is all you have? (You challenge the patient.)

Pt.: Well, it just is—no one else cares about me any more.

Dr.: How's that?

Pt.: Well, Mrs. B., my neighbor, was a real friend, but she died about a month ago and since then, I haven't had anyone but the children.

Dr.: So now you really have no one to spend time with but the children? (Summarizing.)

Pt.: No, Doctor, I don't.

Dr.: And no one else will listen to your problems?

Pt.: Yes, I guess that's about it.

Dr.: Don't you feel that you would enjoy spending time with people other than your children?

Pt.: Yes, I suppose so, but I really don't know many people now. (Pause.) I suppose it would be nice to be among other people, but the children are the only ones I have had for so long.

Dr.: Could it be possible that the children and Mrs. B. are the only ones you have tried to be close to?

Pt.: That might be, but I don't see how things can change.

> **Note:** You can continue with your discussion of the patient's situation. It may be possible for you, since her feelings of loneliness have been brought out in the open, to suggest a course of action for her that will eliminate the frustrating situation

with her family, e.g., civic or church activities, more contact with old friends, if any. You have successfully uncovered the latent content of this lady's problems—the key to relieving her distress. (Go to No. 3.)

3. After Mrs. Monroe leaves, you open the gift she has just given you, and inside is a $100 bill. What is your future course of action about this?

    A.   Accept the gift and say nothing at a later date.

    B.   Send her a note with the money, explaining that you appreciate her consideration, but that her gift is unreasonable by virtue of its excessive amount.

    C.   Write her and explain that you will deduct this amount from her future bills.

    D.   Return the gift at her next appointment, explaining why you are doing so.

    E.   Accept the gift, but mention at her next appointment that it was unreasonably large and that you will not accept any gifts in the future of that magnitude.

Answer A: Accept the gift, say nothing at a later date.

    Note: Why do you want to play the ostrich? Ignoring this gesture will not change the situation in any way for the patient, except that she has now altered the professional relationship. Do you feel you need this offering from the patient or are you hesitant to discuss the $100 bill with the patient?

Answer B: Send her a note with the money, explaining that you appreciate her consideration, but that her gift is unreasonable by virtue of its excessive amount.

    Note: Why is $100 too much? Would $10 have been all right? The important point to consider is the *principle* of the gift, and the mechanism of transference in which the patient is involved by presenting this gift to you.

Answer C: Write her and explain that you will deduct this amount from her future bills.

    Note: This action is good in that you are pointing out to the patient that you cannot accept a *gift* from her, but that remuneration on her part should be on a *business* basis only. If, however, you had not accepted the gift in the first place, you would have avoided this somewhat sticky necessity.

Answer D: Return the gift at her next appointment, explaining why you are doing so.

    Note: D is really quite clumsy and reopens the subject for further argument. This delay would be a fumbling solution to the problem with which you are faced. All this elephantine maneuvering could have been avoided by refusing the gift at her first offer.

Answer E: Accept the gift, but mention at her next appointment that it was unreasonably large and that you will not accept any future gifts of that magnitude.

> **Note:** In what magnitude are you interested—perhaps $50 or $25 instead? She would probably be happy to oblige you. You should have seen through the *reason* she gave you the gift when it was offered.

Comment: Quite understandably, at this point you may be antagonized with this interview. The acceptable selections that were given *did* eliminate the possibility of refusing the gift. They did so, however, to allow you to see what recourses were available in the event you accepted this gift. The circumstances are extremely rare in which the acceptance of gifts from patients is perfectly free and above board. However, this is clearly a case in which acceptance is contraindicated.

The acceptance of a gift such as this and subsequent refusal because of the amount parallels the story of a young couple. The fellow asks the girl, "Would you sleep with me if I gave you a million dollars?" She responds, "Yes, I suppose so." He asks, "Would you do so if I gave you one dollar?" She replies, "Of course not, what do you think I am, a prostitute?" He says, "Well, we've already established that fact—now we're just haggling about the price." The comparison to the gift above should be clear.

There are a few questions you should ask yourself before accepting any sort of a gift or favor from a patient. Among these are the following: How did you provoke this gift? Is it a real act of generosity and admiration, or did you inadvertently signal the need to your patient for this act? In our present culture gifts are not frequently given as a payment but rather as a symbol of love and appreciation. Do you feel a need for the patient to show appreciation? Why do you need this type of ego support?

Other questions to be considered are the following: why does the patient feel a need to alter the professional relationship and why isn't the patient content in his role as a patient?

In the interview you have just worked through the patient wanted to convert the relationship to that of mother and child to control you. Some patients may try to control your feelings about them, or possibly try to evoke benevolence from you.

MRS. DOWLING: a suicidal patient*

This interview was conducted by Hardin M. Ritchey, M.D., a psychiatrist. We are indebted to Dr. Ritchey for adding the introduction along with his critique and comments to this interview.

One of my early teachers made the point many years ago that a history can be two things: (1) a record of the source of information for the future and (2) a therapeutic tool which converts the first hour into a therapeutic process. This is applicable not only to psychiatric histories but to other medical situations as well. The history as provided by the patient gives information that the therapist uses by his method of inquiry, manipulation, and feedback of the material to a therapeutic end. In recent years I have added a third dimension to the initial interview: the negotiation of a treatment contract between the patient and myself regarding how, where, when, and under what terms we will work together.

During the interview I use a printed form that provides a place for the patient's name, address, telephone number, and age; the spouse's or nearest relative's name, address and telephone number, and the name and address of the referring health professional or agency. It is important that the form be dated. In the righthand column, I record the marital status of the patient including the number of times the patient has married, how long he/she was married the first time, and how long divorced, widowed, or separated. The letter indicating the patient's marital status is circled with a number indicating the number of years of each status. Also added to the form is the person's religion, occupation, spouse's or nearest relative's occupation, and if pertinent to my records, the kind of insurance or third-party carrier that may be involved in the eventual contract negotiations. By the time I have completed the information on the history sheet, I have knowledge of the patient's ability to integrate, ability to recall, and, by the patient's facial expression and the manner in which the material is introduced, I have conceptualized the patient's relationship to his/her nearest relative and whether he/she is acquainted with or interested in the type of work the

---

*Hardin M. Ritchey, M.D., Adjunct Professor of Psychiatry, School of Primary Medical Care, The University of Alabama in Huntsville.

spouse does. The record of the marital relationship suggests many things, such as the stability of this individual's activities, his/her ability to pairbond and form lasting relationships, possible incidents of tragedy in the past life, and the possibility of unresolved tension and grief related to separation, divorce, or other loss.

I mark the religion of the individual as a 1, 2, 3, or 4 plus depending upon the frequency of attendance and the intensity of the faith the individual expresses. For instance, if a person is Protestant but doesn't go to church, I record a 1 plus Protestant. A person who goes to church occasionally or to Sunday school is recorded as 2 plus. A person who goes to both church and Sunday school is 3 plus. A person who goes to church every time the church is open is recorded as 4 plus.

The presence or lack of insurance suggests the type of planning the patient does for the future and the level of his/her responsibility.

By the time this preliminary information has been obtained I have a wealth of information about the patient as well as most of a mental status examination.

This recording is of an interview with a patient whom I had seen several years previously and who called asking to be seen again. On the occasion of this interview, the previous contact was sufficiently remote as to make this essentially an initial history demonstrating the aforementioned parts.

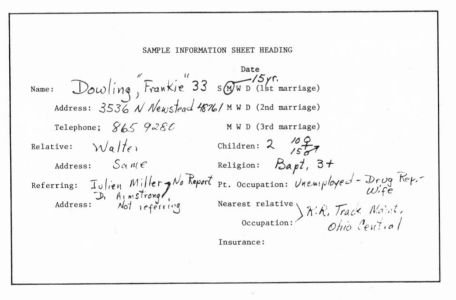

SAMPLE INFORMATION SHEET HEADING

Date

Name: Dowling, "Frankie" 33 S M W D (1st marriage) —/5 yr.

Address: 3536 N Newstead 4876/ M W D (2nd marriage)

Telephone; 865 9280   M W D (3rd marriage)

Relative: Walter   Children: 2 10 9 / 15 8 7

Address: Same   Religion: Bapt, 3+

Referring: Julien Miller—No Report   Pt. Occupation: Unemployed - Drug Rep.-
Dr Armstrong,   Wife
Address: Not referring   Nearest relative / R.R. Track Maint.,
Occupation: Ohio Central

Insurance:

Dr.: Well, let me get some information first. Frankie, is that what your. . .
Pt.: Yes, I am called Frankie.
Dr.: Frankie Dowling.
Pt.: Right, yes sir.
Dr.: How old are you?
Pt.: 33
Dr.: And your address?
Pt.: 3536 North Newstead Avenue.

Dr.: That's a nice place. What's the zip there?
Pt.: 48761
Dr.: And your telephone?
Pt.: 856-9280
Dr.: Who is your family doctor?
Pt.: Dr. Julian R. Miller.
Dr.: Do you want me to say anything to him about your being here?
Pt.: Well, I now go to Dr. Armstrong. I have high blood pressure, which I have always had and Dr. Miller just said he washed his hands of me because almost anything he would prescribe he has to check if it is going to affect my blood pressure so it's just easier. . .

> **Comment:** It is apparent that high blood pressure is a primary issue though not necessarily a basic one. Note that the patient reveals what she has come for very early in the interview. She may later deny this or not come back to it until the very end of the interview. (See p. 154.)

Pt.: Now I asked him, did he not think that I kept fainting continuously and I . . .
Dr.: Fainting?
Pt.: Yes sir, which is my way of hiding as I interpret it. How's that for a little bit of psychology? I bundled up and I fainted. I didn't want to go see Dr. Armstrong and he made me come in for my check-up. And he always wants to put me back in the hospital, which upsets me. And I just wrecked the bike and tore up my hand a couple of weeks ago. I have a motorcycle, and this is not the best thing to do—drive a motorcycle and faint—but every time something comes up that I don't like, that seems to be my way out. Which is not too sharp when you are on a motorcycle, but yet I don't have any control over stopping it. At least I didn't think so until I made a tremendous effort that when I felt myself going I could latch onto something or stop. I haven't fainted since then but Dr. Armstrong said he didn't think I needed to see a psychiatrist. He did suggest that maybe I should take an antidepressant, which I refused to take. I'm not a good patient.

> **Question:** What is the basic issue for this patient?
> A. Not being a good patient
> B. Being in the hospital upsets her
> C. Life or death
> D. She doesn't like the effect of antidepressants
> E. The physician's lack of referral to a psychiatrist

> **Answer:** C. The patient said, ". . . it is not the best thing to do. . ." which means that she recognized the potential for injuring or killing herself by this action. ". . . that seems to be my way out . . . I don't have any control over stopping it." Here she recognizes that when "something comes up that I don't like" my way out is to tempt fate, flirt with death and "I don't have any control" (translated this might read, "I don't choose to take control.") Thus, suicide is the basic or most important issue.

146

At this juncture I elected to return to the introductory material rather than allowing the patient to proceed into information that may require more time to deal with than I am willing to use at this point. It is easy to get distracted in this way and not get an initial contract.

Dr.: So you are saying that there is not much reason to talk to Dr. Miller about your having been here. (Temporarily ignoring the basic issue.)

Pt.: No, he treats me for colds and things like that but as far as any medicine, I see Dr. Armstrong. He is the one who gives it because of my blood pressure, which is . . .

Dr.: Is there any one in particular that you do have or want me to give any report?

Pt.: No sir.

Dr.: Okay, so this is just going to be between you and me, whatever we decide. How long have you been married?

Pt.: Oh, about 15 years.

Dr.: Married one time?

Pt.: Yes sir.

Dr.: You have two children, you say?

Pt.: Yes sir.

Dr.: How old?

Pt.: One will be 15 in February and the girl was 10 in August.

Dr.: And what's your religion?

Pt.: Baptist, narrow-minded Baptist.

Dr.: You go to church?

Pt.: Yes sir, I teach a Sunday school class.

Dr.: You are at least a 3 + Baptist then aren't you?

Pt.: (Laugh.) Foot-washing type, picnic on the grounds type. I teach the 65-year-old ladies and up. They range about in their 80's and 90's mainly.

Dr.: So you are working with those who are about to enter the Kingdom.

Pt.: Well, they are really refreshing. They are a bigger help than trying to talk with someone in your own age group. They are more materialistically interested, which I don't seem to be, for some reason. These little old ladies are so glad to be alive every morning. Which is very refreshing to me.

Dr.: And you are not working now?

Question: This is a leading question. How would you rephrase this question to avoid leading the patient?

Answer: Are you working now?

Pt.: No sir.

Dr.: What's your husband do?

Pt.: He's a gandy dancer railroad worker.

Dr.: Is he working?

Pt.: Yes sir, when I came to you before. . .

Dr.: What's his name?

Pt.: Walter . . . he was a carpenter. (Pause.)

Note: Even though the patient was interrupted, she finished her comment after answering the question.

Dr.: He went from carpenter to gandy dancer, that's quite a step.

Pt.: Well, they're both working with your hands.

Dr.: Yes.

Pt.: You are working or making things and he has a lot of time. He whittles wood objects and things like that.

Dr.: I see.

Pt.: Got a tremendous security factor out there which is important to him.

Dr.: Who does he work for?

Pt.: Ohio Central

Dr.: Oh, I see, so has he got enough seniority to stay pretty good.

Pt.: Ah, yes sir.

Dr.: You had worked for a drug firm as a . . .

Pt.: For 2 years, yes sir.

Dr.: . . . as a field representative.

Pt.: Right.

> **Comment:** The initial information has been completed and the therapeutic process is to be started. It is important to get a contract with the individual about what she wants and is willing to do so that there is a clear understanding on the part of all parties about what is to be done, of my service, and the amount of my fees. This negotiation follows.
>
> One of the dangers of beginning an interview with this type of data gathering is that it is basically a question–short answer (answer only what I ask) interaction. The patient may quickly develop the expectation that all I want from her is short answers and will continue with short answers when I am seeking more information. I am asking to have the patient accept responsibility for giving information while I retain control of the direction and topic to be considered.

Dr.: Well, we talked a little bit the other day, Frankie, about your coming here and what I'm willing to do and where I am. As I told you I am retired, and I don't treat folks anymore, particularly anybody who is into getting into any kind of bad spot, needing hospitalization or ongoing treatment. If they do, I would only be willing to work with them with the understanding that they would arrange to get the kind of care they needed. I'm not willing to assume ongoing responsibility for a couple of reasons. I've done it for many years and very successfully, but now I'm not willing to be tied down to taking care of people everyday and second I'm not in town but about two days a week. I do not think that's an appropriate way to cover a medical practice so I quit practice. What I am doing is working with some people who are interested in changing spots. I've learned some things in the last few years, and I'm willing to work with people in working on some change for themselves. If they are into doing that, and certainly into using what I have available in the way of protection for them and support for them, on the weekends when I'm here. I'm not sending bills now so that the work that I do, I want to be paid at the time I do it. If you have insurance policies or whatever, I'm willing to help you fill them out so you can collect it, but I'm not into collecting from them or processing them. My regular rate is $60 an hour. I am willing to work for less than $60 an hour or more, so that's a negotiable thing. I price myself at $60 an hour. That doesn't mean that I am unwilling to work with someone who is not willing to pay that much or not able perhaps at the time to use that much money for that purpose. So that's where I am, I'm interested in knowing, as I said when we talked this morning, if there is something that you want to work with me on.

Pt.: I thought there should be something changed in me.

Dr.: Okay.

Pt.: And I don't know how to go about doing it because I am not aware when I am doing it. I'm sure that it's not something that my husband has made up, but I just don't understand.

> **Comment:** The patient does not answer the question about the contract and starts out on some of the things that she wants to do. It is important to return to the point and get a contract before continuing. Is she willing to work, to be governed by the limits of what I am willing to do with her?

Dr.: So are you interested in coming and working?

Pt.: Yes.

Dr.: What do you want to do? Do you want to work every week?

Pt.: I don't know.

Dr.: Do you want to call and work when you think you want to?

Pt.: Yes, I think that would . . . it seems to go like a cycle. There might be weeks when I could keep under control and then there might be weeks when everything is just upset. I can't understand why I let them get that way.

> **Comment:** I note at this point she describes her symptoms as cyclic.

Dr.: I'm willing to work with you in whatever way you want to go. In other words, I have given up most of my bad habits insisting that people do something they don't want to do.

> **Comment:** "Whatever way you want to go" refers to the topic and not to the therapeutic procedures or methods.

Pt.: I'm a bad patient to start with.

Dr.: This suits me. What are you willing to pay me?

> **Comment:** I have elected to place her in charge of what she will do and to avoid reinforcing her rebellious position. In transactional analysis language this is called stroking the rebellious child.

Pt.: (Laugh.) how is 50 cents?

Dr.: That's not enough. (Laugh.)

Pt.: Nothing ventured nothing gained. (Laugh.)

Dr.: You'll never get anything unless you ask.

Pt.: That's right. (Laugh.) I learned something in sales anyway. I've taken up throwing papers, which is very fulfilling to me. A lot of people don't seem to understand this but I enjoy talking to people. It's still out in the public and people have all kinds of jobs, all kinds of hobbies, and it's amazing the number of things you can learn from people. I deal mainly in apartments but I make about $50 a month off it, and so I'd be willing to go most of that, how's that?

Dr.: How frequently will you be coming?

Pt.: At least once a month I'm sure. I don't know how bad my problem is. Possibly you would be able to give better direction.

Dr.: Okay, let's do this. I certainly will be willing to see you for $50 and then if you require being seen more than once a month, we'll make some other arrangements for the other time, okay?

Pt.: Right.

Dr.: Alright, that's good enough. (Pause.) Anything you want to know from me now.

Pt.: No sir.

Dr.: About what I'm expecting of you or what I'm offering you or whatever?

> **Comment:** It is important to find out what the patient expects of me so that I can either perform in that manner or define the terms that I am willing to make. An important part of history taking is this point. Misunderstandings between my patients and me develop from not checking out expectations. If I have not clearly defined what the patient wants and what I expect of him/her, then I may have implied agreement to an impossible demand.

Pt.: Well, I'm assuming what you will be able to do is to lead me in a direction where I need the change, so that I'll be able to see and understand why I'm doing some of this, or not necessarily that I have to understand it but at least that I can. That I should be making this change.

Dr.: Okay.

Pt.: I mean, I'm not trying to be unoffensive to everybody because you can't do that but certainly with people I live with.

> **Comment:** This not a good example of a clear contract because she is talking about things that she "should" do. It would have been better to clarify this by saying that, "I am willing to help in considering and developing some new options for your life and in understanding how you have arranged to get to the place that you are and to select what changes you may wish to make in the future." As it reads at this point there is the suggestion that I am going to do more than half of the work by agreeing to lead her in a direction where she "needs" to make a change. Her resultant position will be of an "obedient child" in that she is going to "try" to do what she "should."

At this time a psychotherapeutic intervention can be made in the history-taking. That is to invite the patient to accept ownership of her position. For example: "Hey, are you willing to be in charge of your life?"

Dr.: Let's use our time here and kind of get up-to-date on what's been going on and where you are. I'm distressed to hear you are having blood pressure problems. You are not old enough.

Pt.: I've had them since I was 14.

Dr.: Wow, you've had high blood pressure since 14.

Pt.: Yes, sir. I used to have to take a great deal of medication four or five times a day.

Dr.: How did you arrange to have high blood pressure by 14?

> **Comment:** This is a therapeutic intervention as before. It is her blood pressure. She will own it as part of herself after she accepts responsibility for it as a part of herself.

Pt.: My mother was a really unique person, who recently died. She drove me bananas, and I left home at 13. I was through with high school and had entered college and was out working on my own and my dad offered that if I would come up here, he would pay for my college and I wouldn't have to work. He lived in Baton Rouge and my mother lived in Coral Gables, but they were not divorced at the time. My dad lived in Baton Rouge and ran the business. Then when they got divorced they divided up the money and the house and this type of thing. There wasn't much of a division—mother got just about everything.

Dr.: What kind of business did your dad have?

Pt.: He still has. He deals in small loans. Loan shark is not a word he likes but that is essentially what it is.

Dr.: Uh huh.

Pt.: And this was something my great uncle had started when we all lived with him.

Dr.: Then this was his business. How old was your mother when she died?

Pt.: She was 62.

Dr.: And your father is how old now?

Pt.: He's 65, 66 Christmas.

Dr.: And he's in pretty good health?

Pt.: Oh, he's an alcoholic; he could die at any moment. He goes to Dr. Mirk. He saved him once, when his intestines perforated five or six years ago and he told him then that if he didn't quit drinking that he would die. He has cirrhosis of the liver severely and he's a diabetic now and has eye diseases, typical of an alcoholic. My mother was one also and each of my father's four wives have been alcoholics. He was prone to pick the same type of women that are alcoholics as well. How'd you like to be in the family?

> **Comment:** I could have effectively stroked her at this juncture for not making a gallows transaction, namely the comment, "How would you like to be in the family." In the gallows transaction such a statement is offered as a joke and

151

followed by a laugh, which indicates the tragic, self-destructive nature of the script of her family. An appropriate supportive, therapeutic intervention at this point would have been an empathic remark about the hurt that is covered by her words and the way in which she attempts to pass off tragic family circumstances with a humorous remark.

Dr.: Did you have any brothers?

Pt.: I have one sister.

Dr.: You have *a* sister. Is she older or younger?

Pt.: She's 3 years older than me. She's expecting her fourth child just any second now. She's been married to somebody who's 65.

Dr.: Has she been married several times?

Pt.: This is her second marriage. She left her first husband and her two children and just walked out the door. Took her clothes and said she had had enough about 4 years ago.

Dr.: That's an interesting new decision that she made.

Pt.: She's stronger than I am. I would have never done that if I had wanted to do it. I have never wanted to leave the kids, of course, I've wanted to kill them at times but I've never wanted to leave the kids because they are fun to be with. I'm still that much of a kid, I like to play games and you know, I can play with either one of them.

Dr.: She just decided that she had had enough of everything, uh? Has she talked with you about that?

Pt.: Not really. She asked how would I feel about her marrying this gentleman that was close to Dad's age. He would not be my type of selection, but she had been living with him for a year, so I told her, why don't you just continue living with him? Of course, she doesn't talk much to me because she thinks I'm very religious, which I'm really not, but when you work in the church and you study the Bible people are prone to think that way and that isn't true.

Dr.: She was not?

Pt.: She was afraid I was going to say, "No, you're a naughty girl" and all this, you know. It didn't bother me at all if that's what she wants to do. I've not been in her shoes so I'm not judging her. I'd just rather live with someone than be married because if it didn't work out it would be easier to separate that way. She's happy.

Dr.: So she's getting along okay now?

Pt.: Yes sir. They live where there is water, no outhouse, just a shell of a house, doesn't even have floors, or ceilings. There are just stubs holding it up.

Dr.: Do they live in the country?

Pt.: Well, it's in Marion, outside of Nashville, out in that area. They've got several acres.

Dr.: Does he farm?

Pt.: No, he fixes cars.

Dr.: I see. And she's liking what she's doing now?

Pt.: Yes sir.

Dr.: She really ditched the whole works.

Pt.: She did.

Dr.: What sort of circumstances was she in before?

Pt.: I don't know how to explain it. She had a very nice husband, we thought, and he was good to her as far as we could see. She went out and worked and when her youngest child, she has a boy 13 and one 9, and when the youngest one started to school she went to work. It seems like when she went to work, she couldn't handle the passes that were made at her. She worked at a car lot answering the phone. She did not go to college or anything.

Dr.: You mean by pass, sexual advances that were made?

Pt.: Well, salesmen. But this is a typical thing when you are in sales. Passes are made and they don't mean anything. That's just like saying hello. And she began to take them seriously and so she started dating other people.

Dr.: I see. So this is a thing that she took on seriously rather than as a part of the patter or banter . . .

Pt.: That's the way I view it. I could be wrong, but that's the way . . .

Dr.: That's in your head?

> **Comment:** My last reply is a therapeutic effort in the direction of stroking the patient for and pointing out the fact that she has owned the above information as coming from herself rather than being fact. "That's the way I view it" is her interpretation of where her sister is and how she views her sister's life.

Pt.: Right, because as I see it, I was with salesmen and I see how they are. I think that's what happened, because she started out dating a salesman and one day he promised to marry her and divorce his wife and of course he never did anything.

> **Comment:** I have a picture of the only sister and her circumstances, and I am ready to move on.

Dr.: Have you been in pretty good health aside from your blood pressure problem?

Pt.: Yes sir.

Dr.: Got along all right with your babies?

Pt.: Well, I had blood pressure problems with them but Dr. Miller has always been aware of it and I've been going to him a long time.

Dr.: Have you had any times during your life when you've been upset? I've seen you sometime for some reason, I've forgotten why.

Pt.: Because I want a piano. I didn't have a piano, still can't play it but I take lessons every week. This is the one thing that I pay for out of my paper money. I've talked myself into it. It irritates me no end that I can do it and yet then talk myself out of it. But taking an antidepressant which . . .

Dr.: How often do you have cycles of depression?

> **Comment:** The word "depression" was introduced by me. From the initial exchange around the topic of depression I do not know what the patient means by it. I do know antidepressants have been prescribed and she describes her discomfort as cyclic. Later in the interview the meaning is clarified. (See pp. 154 and 163.)

Pt.:   I judge maybe twice a year.

Dr.:   How long do you keep yourself depressed?

Pt.:   I don't know, they might range from a couple of days to three or four weeks. It seems totally unrelated to anything. But the antidepressant causes you to act like somebody else and . . .

> **Note:** The patient used the word "you" rather than "me." This is evidence that she does not accept ownership for her feelings and thoughts.

Dr.:   You've taken some antidepressants from time to time.

Pt.:   Dr. Armstrong put me on some when I first started going to him. I wrecked the car with the company when I first started with them and I got a skull fracture and a concussion and my blood pressure went 280/160 or something like that.

> **Comment:** This is an important bit of information that she has volunteered in spite of the fact that she did not answer the question. She has made a significant observation of herself. She has episodes of depression and I will use this information along with previously related material to begin a therapeutic formulation. It appears the important issue here is going to be about survival and depression.
>
> The patient early in the interview also made remarks about recent accidents that she had had on a motorcycle. Very early in the history a patient will reveal the basic issue if I allow myself to hear it.

Dr.:   You have a lot of accidents!

Pt.:   Well. (Laugh.)

Dr.:   What's funny? (A confrontation.)

Pt.:   I mean . . .

Dr.:   What's funny about that?

Pt.:   Well, it could be my means of escape.

Dr.:   Yeh, by being dead.

Pt.:   Oh, most definitely. I always when I get depressed . . .

Dr.:   I don't preceive that as being funny.

Pt.:   Well, maybe it isn't. I've done better this time by not getting involved with the suicide tendencies because I realize there is more to life out there.

Dr.:   You've been thinking about killing yourself from time to time?

Pt.:   (Nods "yes.")

Dr.:   When have you been contemplating this last?

Pt.:   Oh, 3 or 4 hours ago.

Dr.:   This recently, uh? (Pause.) How long have you been hurting this badly?

Pt.:   Always.

Dr.:   As long as you can remember.

> **Comment:** Now it is apparent that the issue is one of life and death. This issue is acute. She is deciding whether to kill herself or not. The therapeutic effort is now goal directed to deal with the issue of suicide. Until this is settled—the matter

of survival or taking care of oneself—no other issues can be dealt with in other than a manipulative and unsatisfactory way. The treatment goal is clear and the message is urgent. If she does not resolve this basic issue, there will be no future. All movement from here on is dedicated to a resolution in favor of living.

Pt.: Actually when my mother died. I loved her a great deal, but she was a miserable mother. And the only way I would hate her is because I loved her so much. But she never acted like a mother and she just died very suddenly. She had just turned 62 and three days later the people at the apartment called me and said, "They found your mother," and said, "What do you want us to do with her?" which was a total surprise. She weighed like 200 lbs. and was about 5′ 4″, and she was very large. She had developed some high blood pressure in later life. She had always had low blood pressure before. But evidently she had just had a heart attack in her sleep and passed away. But this was more a sense of release. I didn't feel guilty, and I'm sure I wished her dead as a child many, many times. She threatened to move in here with me and I had to be very firm with myself as well as with her and tell her I couldn't live with her. I guess two women in a kitchen just never work out, but I knew I couldn't live with her. As I said I felt kind of a sense of release, and yet my husband is just like her (laugh) and I can't . . . I criticize my dad for having somebody time after time of the same type and yet I seem to put my dependency feelings with somebody who is of the same type. The only difference is that my husband doesn't drink. (Laugh.)

> **Comment:** These laughs are examples of gallows laughter that I chose not to deal with at this time. They are described by Eric Berne as the "scripty laugh." I see these as less pathologic than the "gallows transaction," in which the issue is death. The laugh reflects the feeling of futility.

Dr.: You mentioned the other day when you talked to me that you and your husband had been having a bad time and that he'd been having troubles and that you've decided that you were going to help him by quitting work or something?

> **Comment:** I am now interested in finding what support she has to call on at home.

Pt.: He seemed to be depressed by me and has continued to be so that he did not want me to work. He wanted me to stay home and I had always felt like my mother was never at home. She was always gone and would hire babysitters until we got to be teenagers or at least until we started high school. I just always wanted to be home with my kids when they started high school and my son started this year.

> **Comment:** This signals that she has been staying alive until her son got into high school. This information again substantiated the idea that she is considering killing herself in the near

future. Previously her attempts at self-destruction have been largely "accidental." However, with this "release date" in her life plan, it may allow more destructive efforts and is possibly the reason that she sought help at this time out of another level of awareness.

Dr.: You wouldn't have been very happy at home with mother anyway?
Pt.: Probably not. I never had that chance to find out.
Dr.: I see.
Pt.: I don't know.
Dr.: So you were involved in using a lot of stuff from the past in your life that didn't have any particular bearing at this time in making some recent decisions.
Pt.: I guess. (Laugh.)
Dr.: Wow!

Comment: This is a therapeutic summary with acceptance that is information accepted with a feeling state (mirth).

Pt.: I like staying at home if I had . . .
Dr.: You want to stay married to this guy?
Pt.: I care a great deal about him.
Dr.: What do you mean?
Pt.: Well, when we split up and he moved into some apartments down the way, it just seemed I'd rather be miserable with him than miserable without him. You know, if you try to weigh the good and the bad, I had rather be with him.
Dr.: Well, would you be willing to feel good either place?

Comment: This reply confronts the patient that she has a choice about feeling good or miserable.

Pt.: I guess I don't really think that's possible.
Dr.: Not really? You never really felt good or don't have permission to feel good?
Pt.: That's the way it is. I don't have permission.
Dr.: Wow.
Pt.: As I said, I'm a purple-headed monster. That's why I said surely there's some way I can change.
Dr.: Is Walter into changing? Or how did you arrange for him to be beating up on you? Or to be around when he was doing that sort of thing?
Pt.: I try not to get him that irritated. I realize that I can get him that irritated. A lot of people can get him that mad, but when I can see the signs coming I try for it not to happen but sometimes explosions happen just very suddenly. This last time I put the towel on the wrong side of the sink and this just exploded him completely.
Dr.: So unless you do things just absolutely right he's going to be pissed off and beat you up?

Comment: I often use vulgarity as a means of giving permission for freer expression and suggesting protection of the patient from my criticism.

Pt.: Yeh (laugh). I don't mean to make him out to be a monster because that's what he's called me, but he just sometimes gets that angry. The only way he knows is to strike with his hands.

Dr.: So are you into leaving him now?

Pt.: No, I don't think I'm strong enough to leave him, but I don't really want to. I'd like to make it where it could be some kind of peace and harmony. I don't really know what I think.

Dr.: But he's not into changing? He's not willing to come to work with you and with me in this situation?

> **Comment:** Again, I used a leading negative phrase rather than, "but is he into changing? Is he willing to come to work. . ."

Pt.: No sir.

> **Comment:** This attempt to have the patient's husband come to work with her as a therapeutic ally is apparently out. Since I asked a leading negative question I am not sure, for the patient may just be agreeing with me rather than giving information. It is important to make clear that my effort will not be on the impossible contract of working with her to change him.

Dr.: I'm not willing to work with you on trying to change him.

Pt.: I'm not trying to change him. I'm just trying to make the situation livable.

Dr.: I'm not even doing that either, because I'm not sure it is.

Pt.: Well, it just seems like things are not right for me, how's that?

Dr.: Right. I'm into working with you on you getting to another spot in your life. I'm impressed with the way you've arranged, the way you continue to get yourself hurt. You're an attractive gal, and here you are kicked around and kicking yourself around and keeping your blood pressure up, falling off motorcycles and . . .

Pt.: I used to worry a great deal about my temper and now I keep a lot of it inside, which I'm sure helps cause the blood pressure go up when I don't particularly like for it to go up. As I said, this time I've been able to keep the blood pressure down. I take a very mild diuretic that lowers the blood pressure. I've argued with him about it. Watching my diet seems to do more than anything to keep the blood pressure down. I'm sure that one of the things that has frightened me is that I realize that when mine reaches as high as it jumps to sometimes, that I could have a stroke, and I feel like with my luck I'd be left like a vegetable, not able to move around or think or anything. I wouldn't like that. Now if it killed me, that would be all right, but that's a risky chance you're taking. So I try to stick to the diet. I don't eat pork, things like this, or eat things with salt on it.

> **Comment:** The patient refers to ". . . the blood pressure . . . mine reaches . . . I could have a stroke . . . it killed me . . ." She accepts ownership at times.

Dr.: Okay.

Pt.: So I see that its my mind that causes it to go up frequently. And

Armstrong kept me in the hospital for a week when I had the auto-mobile accident and ran all the checks and there is nothing physically wrong with me causing the blood pressure to go up.

Dr.: All right. So we're dealing in this situation with your problems and what you've been into over a long period of time. There's one thing I want to negotiate with you today. Are you willing to do a little work now?

> **Comment:** A renegotiation of a therapeutic contract is necessary to see if the patient is willing to work on the identified basic issue. The first ploy in this is to say that she is not certain she can. This is confronted and a contract to work is accepted.

Pt.: If I can. Not certain that I can do it, how's that?

Dr.: I'm certain you can, if you will. Will you?

Pt.: Okay.

Dr.: I'm interested in you getting to a new position with yourself about living. One of the ways that I am unable to deal with you is dead.

Pt.: I don't really think, that I will ever do anything, because I don't like pain at all. It seems like I would have done something quite some time ago. I don't like taking pills, even if I had pills to take that would do it. So I realize that I'm not strong enough to do something about it. It's just something that I think about but I never do anything.

> **Comment:** She does not want to use any of the above methods. However, she does not mention the fact that she has tried accidental death by automobile accident, the motorcycle accident, and that she would like to be dead if she thought she could do it with a stroke and not leave herself paralyzed and dependent. This is an ambivalent position revealing an unacceptable wish to be dependent. She fantasizes a stroke, paralysis, and the need to be cared for. The malignancy of her instruction to be dead and the tragedy and pain resulting from her unwillingness to ask for what she wants reflect her decision that she is not important enough to deserve having her own needs met without serious illness.

Dr.: This has been a conflict for a long time. What I'm interested in at this time is an agreement with you, from you, with yourself that you are going to take care of yourself here and now and you are not going to kill yourself. That is, not only that you are not going to kill yourself but that you are going to live and you are going to learn to have a good time and do some other things and not arrange to have somebody else to kill you. Say some crazy nut.

Pt.: (Laugh.) I've thought about that. Mother tried her best, I think, to drive me crazy. I think she frequently did a bang up job except at 13 I seemed to have had more gumption because I just walked out and left her. Because I realized what she was trying to do, and she never missed me one way or the other and probably that would be so with Walter or almost anybody. Cooking and housecleaning is not very thrilling to me. I can tolerate it and do it if that's what it's going to take, but somewhere along the line I have to have another out. I don't know particularly what that is, but I've decided after the last fall that I wasn't going to do that anymore and I haven't. I haven't fainted one time since I wrecked on the bike. It didn't wreck the bike at all, but it just seemed like because I didn't want to go see Dr. Armstrong that was my way of getting out of it.

Dr.: I'm aware of the fact that getting out of things in that way can be a very terminal sort of thing and I'm not willing to work with you on being dead. I want to work with you alive.

> **Comment:** Any effort to work with the patient on any issue other than being alive is in fact acquiescing to and going along with her initial instructions to kill herself and to be dead. Until the issue of being alive is positively agreed to, any other work is detrimental to the therapeutic process by discounting the basic life-and-death issue.

Pt.: I'm trying, you know that.

Dr.: That's not where I want to be, I'm not willing to try. So get in touch now with your sadness.

Pt.: When Walter and I separated, I felt so dreadful. (Crying) I felt like the only thing that would make everybody happy would be that if I would leave or just kill myself and then people would have the benefit of the life insurance or whatever. And I have a cousin that I've not been very close to but someone that I admire a great deal, a very intelligent man. He's in his early 40's and he at that time was living in Detroit. He teaches at Western University. He has several Ph.D.'s and a law degree, all kinds of things. I don't know what all he does but I spoke with him on the phone and he sent me a plane ticket to fly to Detroit, which I did within the hour. I guess it was in February because it was St. Patrick's Day when I got in. They had a huge parade that they celebrated, the Mayor and everything, and he took me to the art museums and things that I never had an opportunity to see. Of course I had really not been out of the South except to go to Pittsburgh in training with the company. And I did almost nothing but work up there. There's not a whole lot to see in Pittsburgh in itself anyway. This was very exciting and I realized there was another way of life and that you could have fun, but when I came back home it just kind of all washed away. I regret that I'm not strong enough to keep that feeling instilled in me. I seemed to feel that I can't do anything right, everything always coming out wrong. Of course, I've got a lot of people telling me how wrong I do things so this doesn't help. People I should learn to tell to drop dead I seem to listen to them.

> **Comment:** There is an important bit of information in this paragraph that I would note for future use. The patient has a cousin in Detroit who is interested in her. If her marriage comes apart or she finds herself alone and unable to cope with her destructive tendencies, he may be an effective person to offer her aid.

The therapeutic effort and tempo is picked up at this time—to achieve a contract to live. Subsequent interventions are confronting the discounts and the rationalizations that are used by the patient to avoid owning her self-destructive goals, accepting responsibility for change, and agreeing to live.

Dr.: Are you willing to listen to yourself instead of other people?

Pt.: Yeh, but I don't do it.

Dr.: I'm interested in you being alive and having a good time for yourself rather than for other people.

Pt.: Never thought about it. I don't really know what I would like to do. I've always tried to do things for other people. I don't really know why. After all this much time, and as much schooling and all, it looks like I ought to be able to come up with something. (Pause.)

Dr.: So at the present time what you are living for is other people. (Pause.)

Pt.: I guess so.

Dr.: If you could stay around with a lot of people who, uh, beat you up periodically pretty soon you could have reason enough to knock yourself off, huh?

Comment: This is an example of collecting bad experiences until the patient has enough to justify her suicide.

Pt.: Well, being with him this long, uh, and doing it, It's like I said, I don't really think I would ever do it. I'm sure that a lot of people say that it's like being an alcoholic. You can quit at any time and yet they really can't. I'm sure that sometime I might try to do something, but since I've never tried anything, I don't feel that's really a risk.

Dr.: So, what are you going to do? (Pause.) Are you willing to take care of yourself?

Pt.: I don't really know how. (Pause.) If I knew how, then possibly I wouldn't be where I am now.

Dr.: One of the ways to take care of yourself is to not kill yourself and not to get someone else to do it and not have an accident on your motorcycle, with your automobile or get run over by a truck. All of these things are ways in which you can take care of yourself. Would you be willing to take care of yourself?

Pt.: Evidently, since I haven't done anything so far.

Dr.: I'm aware of the fact that you haven't taken care of yourself up to now.

Pt.: It's like I said, I just don't know what I'm supposed to be doing.

Comment: This is a plea on the part of the patient from a victim position to place the responsibility on someone to teach her all the things that she is supposed to do while she proceeds on her self-destructive course. It is important that the interviewer recognize this as a trap and not elect to support this course.

Dr.: So, you are not willing to take care of yourself until you have learned all the things you are supposed to be doing?

Pt.: (Laugh) Well, I'm taking care of myself, in a way.

Dr.: You came to see me. I agree with that. I want you to take care of yourself when I'm not around.

Comment: The patient continues to avoid the issue.

Pt.: For one thing, it's staying at home. I found that a lot of things that I used to think were important turned out to be, things that are NC (nobody cares). This John Coston, on the radio, who talks about things being NC said, "I find that like you don't get all the clothes ironed at this time; well, that's really not so dramatic, you know. There's tomorrow, next week, and it's really an NC." Now, if I take things very slowly and not put so much emphasis on things, almost everything is NC. It really doesn't matter and yet we rationalize things that way. To my way of thinking, living is an NC.

Dr.: You don't matter?

Pt.: (Laugh.) That's right. There's only a point to which you can try to do it, but taking things slowly has helped, at least, I don't seem to get upset as much inwardly and maybe that's why I've been able to keep my blood pressure down.

Question: What does the patient's laugh mean?

Answer: I don't know. Hopefully, she may have recognized the fact that she places herself in an "I don't count" transactional position.

Dr.: Even if you do get upset, are you willing to take care of yourself?

Pt.: Well, I'm trying. I called to see if I couldn't do something to make a change somewhere.

Comment: *Trying* is the way in which people don't do things, and this was placed along with the negative statement "to see if I can't do something," rather than "if I *can* do something." I missed this, and I consider it a therapeutic mistake. It is not necessary or possible to confront every such statement in the history of a patient. However, I do consider that a statement of how she will not change could have been confronted therapeutically. As it turns out, I bought it; I agreed that she couldn't. This is the result of having an idea in my head that her feelings needed to be identified before going to a more positive contract. This illustrates the danger of being preoccupied with what I've got in my head instead of listening to what the patient is saying and hearing the message.

Dr.: And so you couldn't and what are you going to do? (pause).

Pt.: Keep struggling, I guess.

Dr.: And feel how?

Pt.: Like I always have. I don't see another way of feeling since I've felt this way all along. I just don't understand how I'm supposed to feel.

Dr.: Are you into living?

Pt.: Yes. There should be more to life than what I'm getting out of it. I felt like maybe I should be putting more into it.

Dr.: Are you willing to live no matter what? (Pause.)

Pt.: I don't know. I don't know if I'm strong enough. It's like I said. What few people that I did share with felt that I should leave Walter—that this would be the best thing for me. Get a job and do something else and leave him—that there are other fish in the ocean type thing, but I don't know that I'm strong enough.

Dr.: I'm not into your leaving Walter or staying with him. I am into your being alive and so that's where I'm staying.

Pt.: I don't really see that anything I've done has been worthwhile to keep living for, and until I see something I am able to do that's worthwhile, I don't understand . . .

Dr.: Would you be willing to be worthwhile just as a person without doing anything?

Pt.: Yeh, that would be . . .

Dr.: I think that you are a nice person. I love you as a person whether you did anything or not.

> **Comment:** Note her change to a child-like feeling position after this supportive and nourishing intervention. She will not make a firm commitment to life when she is not in such a feeling state.

Pt.: I think this is what my cousin emphasized to me. (Crying.) He didn't really care what I had done or what I was fixing to do (crying) which is kind of unusual. Nobody in my family has ever thought that way. My mother always pitted my sister and me against each other. If we got too close, she would tell lies to one or the other so that we would constantly stay at odds. As long as she had us that way we would not join forces and tell on her, more or less, what she was doing, and the different men that would come around and all. We would never tell our father, and even now my sister and I are not very close and we will never be very close. And I'm sure my sister always kind of wants to know what have you done for me recently—not just forever, but recently. There is only so much you can do recently for her. And my dad is just out in left field. He hasn't been to work in 8 or 9 weeks. He's been on the bottle so heavy, but he just really doesn't exist much. His opinions, at least, don't really affect me very much. So I'm back to listening to Walter and I think I don't seem to do anything right, which is a drawback. It's kind of hard to keep self-confidence that you are a person even.

Dr.: Yeh.

Pt.: When you don't do anything right.

Dr.: Are you willing to just be? (Pause.)

Pt.: I'd like to try it but I don't. It looks awful far away. (Pause.) It's like learning to play the piano and when you make mistakes just keep playing and think next time when I play maybe I won't make that mistake instead of stopping and going back and playing the right note which ruins the whole piece. And frequently people can't tell that you played the wrong note anyway. It's very hard to keep playing on the piano, which is kind of what you are saying. Just to keep life going even though mistakes happen. Just to keep going and keep thinking that you will get through the piece anyway, and still be thought of as being able to play, which is kind of the way in which I am viewing life. That even though I make mistakes with it, just to keep going and not dwell on the one thing that upsets me at the time.

Dr.: Will you do that?

Pt.: Well, I told you I don't play the piano very well. And I've been trying for . . .

> **Comment:** Again the word "trying" rather than "I have decided to. . ."

Dr.: I'm not interested in your playing the piano. I'm interested in your being alive. (Pause.)

Pt.: Well, I keep trying to play the piano, so evidently I keep trying to want to stay alive, too.

Dr.: Are you willing to be alive whether you play the piano or not?

Pt.: Yes, I learned quite some time ago that I would never learn to play the way I would like to play.

Dr.: I'm quite willing to agree to that, but I'm interested in hearing what you have to say about living. (Pause.) Are you willing to live for you?

Pt.: I keep saying I never have so I don't understand how to even start off doing it. It's like going into the kitchen and saying I'll make something for me, while at lunch time I just don't even fix anything. I just continue working around the house and I don't even know how.

> **Comment:** A good example by the patient of "trying."

Dr.: Will you learn how?

Pt.: I can try.

Dr.: I know how, will you learn how?

Pt.: (Laugh.)

Dr.: Huh?

Pt.: Yes, I think that's one of the reasons why I called because the last time I did see you I was quite impressed about how content you were with life and accepting the way things were going and not being overly concerned, which seems to be the way I am and having a teenager. They are cause to make you think you are doing everything wrong anyway. They don't like anything, you know. You iron the shirt wrong or iron the wrong shirt, or you have supper at the wrong time. It's inconvenient for them.

Dr.: Are you willing to take care of yourself and live no matter what? If supper is wrong for teenagers for the next 40 years or not?

> **Comment:** Continued evasion of the question is now quite apparent. Were the issue of lesser stature than life-and-death I cease to work on an impasse when the patient is avoiding further effort.

Pt.: I think this is why this concerns me. I suddenly realized that it won't really be long before the kids are gone, and then what am I going to do? (Pause.) If I'm going to eventually end up alone, which is sort of the way I feel now even though I am with the children, when they really do go, where will I be? I am concerned about the future because it doesn't look very bright right now. It looks kind of grim and I'd like to change that. I'd like for it to be another color.

Dr.: Part of the future is being alive. (Pause.)

Pt.: (Crying.) I guess my argument is: look how many people I could make happy by being dead.

Dr.: Who would you make happy by being dead besides your mother?

Pt.: Well, I feel like the kids and Walter most assuredly. And he could have money and do whatever he wanted to do. The money seems to be a bit of a pressure now, and he always resented that I made more money than he did when I was working. I don't guess there's anybody that would make much difference if I were alive or dead really. My dear little ladies in my Sunday school class would say, "Too bad," but that is about the extent of it. As you can see, I'm not learning a whole lot from what they are giving up because they are always so happy to be alive from week to week, day to day. Even though they have, I'm sure, the same problems.

Dr.: So at the present time your position has to do with being dead because you think Wally would like it.

> **Comment:** The use of the word "Wally" here is a therapeutic error and has to do with an association in my head about a former associate involved in some personally damaging business negotiations. This is evidence of the way in which unrecognized and suppressed hostility can break through in an unguarded moment.

Pt.: Well, he and the kids are about the only family I've got that offer any form of caring.

Dr.: But as you are saying they are caring just because you'd leave them some money.

Pt.: Which shows that I'm not really worth very much.

Dr.: In whose head?

Pt.: In mine. (Pause.) I regret sometimes I'm not more religious, and that I could feel death would be a wrong thing to think about, but it doesn't bother me at all. (Crying.)

> **Comment:** The frequency of crying in the interview has picked up as the emotional content escalates with persistence in working on being alive. This escalation often is misinterpreted by the interviewer as being the result of persistence and he/she blames him/herself for causing the patient's discomfort. In fact the professional is revealing the pain and as this begins to surface, the patient is experiencing the pain as sadness. It is now that comforting, positive stroking, and holding can be effective in getting a binding contract to live. Contracts that are made in the "should" and "reasonable" states do not have the binding properties of those made in the "reasonable" combined with the "feeling" state. It is gut feeling that goes with real committment.

Dr.: When did you decide that you would probably kill yourself? Do you remember?

Pt.: I don't remember much before I was eight. Very few things. I seemed to have hated my great aunt then. I don't remember, at least, in my conscious mind at all. I have seen pictures of her. I don't remember at all. I can remember the day they laid her out in the dining room. I don't remember her, I can see a shadow of her, and I can remember what she smelled like. Everything from day one goes from there.

Dr.: What did you decide when she died?

Pt.: I don't remember deciding anything. It's just that I never was very worthwhile even when she was alive. She was prone to care more for my sister.

Dr.: What did she smell like?

Pt.: She smelled like desert flowers. It was a fragrance she wore. And I can remember that smell.

Dr.: Did you like that smell?

Pt.: Not particularly. I have allergies and almost all colognes and alcohol break me out so I don't really wear very much. Most of them kind of make me sick anyway when I smell them for very long. She always seemed to smell this way, at least, what I can remember of her. But I don't remember deciding anything when she died. My mother went absolutely wild. She was wild before that, but then there was no one to pamper her. I guess that's when my mother really left my sister and me. We just had a series of people who took care of us. (Pause.)

Dr.: What are you in touch with now?

Pt.: A purple-headed monster. It just gets bigger and bigger.

Dr.: Will you be willing to work with the purple-headed monster?

Pt.: Yes.

Dr.: Okay.

> **Comment:** I have a therapeutic contract with this patient. She has agreed to work and now I will work with her to help get her in touch with the part of herself that she has designated as the purple-headed monster. Ordinarily, Gestalt therapy is not used in the initial history. However, the suicide issue at hand is of such importance that I am making every effort to clear away obstacles to her giving herself permission to live.

Dr.: What kind of trouble are you having with the purple-headed monster?

Pt.: I don't understand why it's there.

Dr.: Are you the purple-headed monster? Will you be the purple-headed monster and sit over here and tell Frankie what's wrong with her?

Pt.: (Crying.) I don't know what's wrong with her.

Dr.: Be the monster and sit over here and tell her what's wrong with her.

Pt.: I guess I don't have any self-confidence.

Dr.: Get over here and be the purple-headed monster.

Pt.: I'm sitting in the right chair, this one's green.

Dr.: Be the purple-headed monster. Who do you want to be there? Do you want to be Frankie there?

Pt.: (Crying.) I don't know what Frankie is really like.

Dr.: This is what you are telling the monster?

Pt.: That's right, for the monster to go away.

165

Dr.:   Well, tell the monster to go away.

Pt.:   But the monster doesn't, but other people go away.

Dr.:   Tell her, she's sitting right there. There she is. Tell her. (Pause.)

Pt.:   Could be like my nightmare I had as a child. When I get upset frequently it comes back. It's not really a nightmare because it's just before I go to sleep, and I no longer sleep at all anymore. And I learned not too long ago that if I could just say now wait a minute, I'm going to think about daisies and sunshine and the nightmare goes away. That all these years I suffered with these crazy things.

Dr.:   Are you going to work with this purple monster or not?

> **Comment:** I am operating as a gatekeeper of the contract by having the patient either work as she agreed to do or to decide not to work. In either case to have the patient be honest with herself and with me.

Pt.:   I'm trying. (Crying.) I'm honestly trying.

Dr.:   Will you tell the purple monster where you are?

Pt.:   Okay. I'm going to make a move in the right direction, even though I don't know what direction that is and make the purple-headed monster go away never to arise again.

Dr.:   Well, how are you going to take care of yourself?

Pt.:   Well, I'm going to try to stay busy, so I don't think. How's that?

> **Comment:** Again the patient is only willing to try. She is not willing to decide to stay busy.

Dr.:   I don't know. Sit over here and be the purple monster and tell her how you are going . . .

Pt.:   Well, that doesn't work because even if I stayed busy and everybody comes in and blasts me, then the purple-headed monster comes in.

Dr.:   Would you sit over here?

Pt.:   Okay.

Dr.:   And be the purple-headed monster, and tell Frankie how you are really going to cause a row.

Pt.:   That's right, just for me to go home.

Dr.:   Now tell her.

Pt.:   Well, that's the way it is. The minute I go home it will all start.

Dr.:   Yeh, you tell her. Be the monster and tell Frankie.

Pt.:   Well, that's what I just did. The minute I go back and get in the car and drive home . . .

Dr.:   As soon as I get you in the car, I'll teach you. Okay, what else?

Pt.:   Well that's what I need to learn is how to tell the purple . . .

Dr.:   Now one of the ways you're keeping yourself screwed up is you are not keeping your identity straight. When you are in this position, would you be the purple monster, and when you're there, you be Frankie. Are you willing to do this?

Pt.:   Yes, I've done it unconsciously with the children. When the children are not around, I'm not Mama, but when the children are there, I've got the hat on that says, "I'm Mama."

Dr.:   So deal with your monster. Your monster is going to screw you over good. Now when you get in your car, what have you got to say about that, Frankie? Move over there and be Frankie please.

Pt.: I'm going to think about sunshine and daisies and nice yellow things that will be bright and happy, instead of dreary. It's funny, my sister used to have a car that color of purple. My mother had one of another shade that was atrocious. I always hated both of them. I don't know why. I wasn't old enough to drive. I could drive. I used to steal mother's car, but maybe that's why I call myself the purple-headed monster.

Dr.: Will you tell the purple-headed monster how you are going to take care of yourself?

Pt.: Well, by not thinking about the purple-headed monster and when someone else causes the purple-headed monster to come up, I'm going to try to make it turn out to be right instead of wrong even if it ends up hurting the other person.

Dr.: Will you tell the purple-headed monster you're not going to kill yourself no matter what?

Pt.: I never really thought that was a problem. It's why I can't take it very seriously, since I never thought I had enought guts to do it. So, it doesn't seem like that's very important to me. It's like somewhere Frankie is going to take over before the purple-headed monster really does anything.

Dr.: I'm aware of the fact that you won't do that.

Comment: This is her impasse beyond which she is unwilling to go.

Pt.: I won't do what? That I won't kill myself? I haven't.

Dr.: No, I'm aware of the fact you won't say that you're not going to. I'm aware of the fact that you immediately tell me about the ways in which it's not going to happen and how you haven't in the past and all other kinds of bull except one simple thing.

Pt.: Well, I guess, it's like I might break my word.

Dr.: You won't say it.

Pt.: No, I might break my word.

Dr.: Now, I'm aware of that, and I'm not willing to work with you on the basis of getting to a bad enough point where you can knock yourself off.

Pt.: I guess I'm going to have to see a lot more to look forward to.

Dr.: So, you are not willing at this time to say you are going to live no matter what?

Pt.: I could say it, but I'm not all that sure that I would hold up to it. I mean, in all honesty, if I'm not at least honest with myself, then I'm not going to be able to help myself.

Dr.: Okay. Now really where I am on this is: I'm not willing to work with you until this is settled. Because I think if you have not really decided to live and take care of yourself and to not kill yourself, I'm not willing to work with you on getting that done, because that's what you're into doing until that is decided. You understand what I'm saying?

Pt.: I thought I had made that decision but evidently I haven't.

Comment: At this juncture a person might elect to go for a conditional contract. If I were seeing this patient and going to continue to treat her. I would get her to agree to live for 5 years from now or 2 years from now or, if necessary, until Christmas. Limited contracts are tricky. It is important to remember that when the contract limit runs out, the patient may feel relieved of the "obligation" to remain living. It is a hazardous option unless the therapist is willing to assume responsibility for keeping track of such limited contracts and to arrange for negotiation of either a longer, more on-going contract to live or an unconditional contract to live.

Dr.: So then until that day and time, I think you should be in the hospital.
Pt.: (Crying.) No. Hospitals frighten me!
Dr.: This is the way in which you frighten yourself, by being in the hospital. I have difficulty understanding why that's a frightening arrangement when you are considering killing yourself.

Comment: It is apparent that the patient is using being frightened of the hospital as a way to discount her life in terms of her fear; that is, she will not go to the hospital, she continues to consider destroying herself. Since she will not make a therapeutic contract to live and she is unwilling to make the effort to work with effective therapeutic techniques, she is suitable for treatment only in the protected setting of a hospital psychiatric unit. She will require more than casual or parttime treatment. It is now apparent that the defining of the limits of my practice at the beginning of the history-taking was most appropriate. It would be difficult to explain at this time that I am not willing to undertake on-going treatment after I find that this "part-time" patient has become a "full-time" job.

Pt.: I've only been in to have the children and then this one time with Armstrong. Otherwise I've never been in the hospital, so I don't know why either. I had no difficulty having the children.
Dr.: Will you work with somebody else?
Pt.: I don't think so.
Dr.: Well, I'm just not willing to be over that barrel with you. I'm not willing for you to come here and work and get to a bad spot. What I've perceived you're into doing is getting to the spot where you can knock yourself off, and I'm not willing to work with you on getting to that.
Pt.: Okay.
Dr.: I won't do it. Cause I think you're a neat gal and could do a lot for yourself.
Pt.: I have every faith in the psychiatrists that I have come in contact with.
Dr.: I know a young man here who has just come to town whom I like. I think he's perhaps a person you might see and see what you think about him. He's Dr. Bevans. Do you know him?
Pt.: No sir.
Dr.: Would you be willing to see him?
Pt.: Not right now. (Pause.) I guess I just need to talk more with myself and when I can come to that decision then . . .

Dr.: You know, you're not aware of the fact that you don't have permission to think very much of yourself at this time and what I see you into doing is laying up enough reasons to where you can do yourself in. I'm not willing to be a party to that and you won't take the position. You won't give the option of saying you are going to, that you're not going to do it. So what I hear you doing is enlisting my help in helping you get it done. I ain't going to be there.

Pt.: I hadn't looked at it that way.

Dr.: I'm interested in helping you live and I'm interested in helping you have a good time, and I'm interested in you as a person, but I'm not going to work with you on being dead. To blow your middle cerebral out with your blood pressure, or fall off a motorcycle, or getting so upset that you are not going to control yourself or whatever else you could arrange.

Pt.: Okay.

Dr.: Do you understand what I'm talking about?

Comment: At this time the interview may be concluded. The therapeutic interventions have been unsuccessful in gaining a contract for life. However, the patient is aware of the impasse, advised of the gravity of her situation, and has been urged to seek intensive treatment.

Pt.: Yes sir. (Pause.) Yes sir. I just don't dwell about death like that. I guess I just didn't realize that I do think about it maybe more than what I'm admitting to myself.

Dr.: Now, I'm not interested in dwelling about death either. I'm interested in talking about living.

Pt.: If I can come to grips with that and learn to say that . . .

Dr.: I'm not into learning to say that, will you learn to be that? How will you do this?

Pt.: I don't know. Give it a good try though.

Dr.: Yeh, how are you going to try? Are you aware of what trying is?

Pt.: I thought I was. Am I supposed to try and pitch it (thoughts of death)?

Dr.: Try, try and throw that kleenex to me. No, *try* to throw that to me. That's throwing it to me.

Pt.: Oh, just try and not let it go.

Dr.: Right. You see what trying is? All this trying stuff is bullshit. That's how you lie to yourself about what you are really going to do. I'm going to try. I'm going to try means I ain't going to do it. I'm just going to try and try and try.

Pt.: All right.

Dr.: So I'm not willing to accept try. If I'm dumb enough to accept that kind of a con, then I'm working with the purple monster here on getting you dead. You understand what I'm saying?

Pt.: Yes sir.

Dr.: Then what do you do with the "yes sir"?

Pt.: I was just not aware that I'm that suppressed, that the purple-headed monster controls so much.

Dr.: That's the part of you that really hasn't decided to let you live yet. Hey, have you got anything to say to him yet?

169

Pt.: Not right now. I might as well leave. (Pause.) I've got to make more sunshine and daisies, like I said, instead of, I didn't say try, I said that I, instead of letting the purple-headed monster take over. But I agree. Until I learn to push him back there's no point.

Dr.: Yeh, I'm not into that at all. What I'm into is whether you are going to kill yourself or not. And I want to hear you say you're going to live no matter what.

Pt.: Such a simple thing to say. (Pause.) I just don't seem to have a reason. The purple-headed monster is still in control.

Dr.: Whose monster is it?

Pt.: It's my monster. I don't like the monster.

Dr.: Tell him you don't like him. (Pause.) He's already told you what he's going to do to you.

Pt.: I guess he scared me, or else I wouldn't have asked for help. Cause I realized I wasn't strong enough . . .

Dr.: Hey, you're asking for help. You're not asking to get well.

Pt.: What's the difference?

Dr.: There's a hell of a lot of difference between getting well and just going on and having a bad time by getting help so that I can postpone a catastrophic circumstance.

Pt.: I just never had another kind of life. I don't see how you can expect me to feel if there isn't another kind of life.

Dr.: I don't expect you to. Are you aware that other people have a different kind of life?

Pt.: Not really.

Dr.: Oh?

Pt.: The few people I come in contact with don't seem to be enjoying life that much except my sister. She's the only one that I could say is happy. She's actually happy; at least I feel she is. It's not the things she says. It's just the way she acts that you know. I know that she's perfectly content that this is what she likes.

Dr.: How long are you willing to stay alive?

Pt.: During the holidays. (Which are 10 weeks away.)

Dr.: This year? (Pause.)

Pt.: I don't really like Christmas because I never had enough money to give people what I'd like to get them. But I guess everybody always felt that way. But it's very upsetting to me. (Crying.) My mother would come sometimes and Dad would like to come over with his current wife, and it was always a matter of juggling the two of them around because they both wanted to watch the kids open presents. It was just a big hassle and maybe this year there won't be that much of a hassle about everything. So that's kind of something to look forward to.

Dr.: Okay. Well, I'm going to be away in December. I'm going to be doing some work in Texas and I'm going to Hawaii for awhile. I want you to do some work and I think you are a neat gal and I think you can do a lot of work. I just think you are going to. I think it is necessary for you to be in touch with somebody who is going to be closer at hand than I am. If you're as you are into not being willing to make a commitment to be alive, because there's not any way I can be of help to you when I'm in Chattanooga or Huntsville or Murpheesboro or someplace like that. I'm just not willing to have you down here by yourself without that kind of decision. Namely, that you are willing to live.

Pt.:   Well, I appreciate your pointing out the problems to me anyway.

Dr.:   Will you let me hear from you?

Pt.:   Yes sir. (Pause.)

Dr.:   Wait a minute. Will you take care of yourself?

Pt.:   Yes sir.

Dr.:   No matter what?

Pt.:   Yes sir.

Dr.:   You're very valuable.

> **Comment:** No further progress was made after the suggestion that the interview should be concluded. A secondary contract to take care of herself was stroked with reinforcement of the value and of the patient as a person and reinforced with a physical embrace.

MR. MARSHALL: a crisis intervention

The crisis intervention interview is intended to be both diagnostic and therapeutic. The behavior of the therapist is characterized by actively intervening and directing the interview, by giving prompt feedback, and by being honest and open in the expression of his reactions. The crisis interview is one of the most difficult to conduct in that it demands alertness and perceptiveness on the part of the interviewer.

Crisis intervention is usually carried out in one session or in a few brief sessions. The focus is on the here, the now, and the immediate past as it directly relates to the problem. Though it is not a rigid and fixed sequence, the following process usually takes place in the order given:

1. Focusing on the patient's conflict.
2. Focusing on and empathizing with the dominant feeling about the situation.
3. Reviewing the physician's understanding of the situation as a form of feedback.
4. Stating clearly what the physician can offer the patient.
5. Confronting the patient with the need to make plans.

The example of a crisis interview that follows was conducted by Dr. Thomas N. Rusk.* The interview was videotaped in a Veterans' Hospital admission area with prior permission of the patient. This was Dr. Rusk's first contact with the patient for the purpose of evaluating the patient's request for help.

This interview is an illustration of the use of an actively directed, efficient interview using the techniques taught in this manual. The interview demonstrates how nondirective techniques may be controlling and how at the same time the patient is allowed to function in the adult ego state. By this we mean that the patient is able to assert himself, to tell his history, and to feel that he is respected and encouraged to take responsibility for his own future.

Dr.: You came up here for what now?
Pt.: See, about 10 days ago . . . I . . . began hurting.

*San Diego, California.

Dr.: Hurting? Ten days ago.

> **Comment:** A reflection—a direct question about how it hurts might have limited the interview to the hurt, which was tangential to the problem.

Pt.: So then, I went and got me some booze.
Dr.: Yeah!
Pt.: That relieved it (the pain) awhile.
Dr.: Yeah. Do you have a Kleenex?

> **Comment:** This question seems irrelevant, but it is a way of focusing upon the patient's immediate feeling.

Pt.: Oh! I got an old hankie, back here. (The patient gets his handkerchief from his hip pocket.)
Dr.: Okay.
Pt.: And I . . . see, that relieves it awhile.
Dr.: Your eyes are tearing a great deal; you're feeling very sad, or is this tearing for another reason?

> **Comment:** This confrontation forces the patient to look at his feelings.

Pt.: And then . . .
Dr.: Are you feeling very sad right now?
Pt.: No. No. No, hell, I feel fine.
Dr.: Why the tears?

> **Comment:** The doctor confronts the patient's denial. One of the first steps of a crisis interview is to focus on the patient's dominant feelings at the moment.

Pt.: I don't know.
Dr.: Must be feeling pretty sad, don't you think?

> **Comment:** The physician needs to be confident that he is correct before being this direct with a patient, although by adding the question "don't you think?" the directness was reduced.

Pt.: No, I feel all right. But they just come.
Dr.: How long has that been going on?
Pt.: Couple days.
Dr.: Do you think there might be something you're pretty sad and depressed about, that you are trying to hide?
Pt.: Well, it . . . no, I think . . . I don't have any sad feelings. I just feel sorry for myself.
Dr.: Yeah, okay.

> **Comment:** The response shows some acceptance of the patient's position and is a mild reward for recognizing a feeling.

Pt.: What an ass I've made out of myself.
Dr.: What do you mean?

Comment: A focusing question to enourage the patient to say more.

Pt.: It's . . . everything I've ever done in my life is turned out wrong. (Crying.)

Dr.: Okay, so you are feeling pretty angry and sad and depressed.

Comment: The anger detected in the patient's voice is reflected back as a part of the feedback.

Pt.: Well now, don't try and make me think I am . . . I, I'm not.

Dr.: It's clear you are.

Pt.: Well . . .

Dr.: It's clear that you are.

Pt.: I, I . . . I'm down on myself, I, I, don't have anything against nobody.

Dr.: I didn't say you were. All I was talking about was how sad you are.

Comment: Since the patient denies many feelings, the interviewer sticks to sadness, which is easier to acknowledge than anger.

Pt.: And uhh . . . dammit anyway. (Snuffles.)

Dr.: Sounds like you think it's wrong to cry or to be sad.

Pt.: Oh, no, it's not wrong to cry.

Dr.: You sure are fighting it . . . you sure are fighting it. It's okay. It's okay to cry. Go ahead! Leave it out, leave that thing out (referring to the handkerchief).

Pt.: I'll get it back out.

Dr.: Okay. Now, tell you what. Tell me what the situation has been for the last few weeks. What's been going on, who you live with, what the home situation's been like. Everything!

Comment: Step two in the crisis intervention is to focus upon the last few weeks. Multiple questions are used here to encourage the patient to tell his story rather than just answering each question one at a time.

Pt.: Well . . . I told you I was an alcoholic.

Dr.: Yeah, you told me you were an alcoholic.

Pt.: Did I tell . . . I use to live in Evansville. I left there in 1949. I went down there . . .

Dr.: No, no. Now you're talking about '49.

Comment: The physician interrupted the patient to focus him back on the recent events in his life.

Pt.: Well, well . . .

Dr.: I want you to talk just about the last few weeks.

Pt.: All right, so I come back here 4 months ago.

Dr.: Okay, okay, now we're on the track.

Comment: The physician actively rewards the patient for returning to the current problem.

Pt.: I ran into this brother-in-law and sister-in-law, brother-in-law and his wife. You know, they lived in a damned hole there, so I thought, well,

	I'll help them out. I got a job, I got money in my pocket. So I rented a house, I bought myself $700 worth of furniture.
Dr.:	Uh huh.
Pt.:	Now I said that I'm moving out of here.
Dr.:	You were living with them for a while.
Pt.:	Yeah, so I says you can move with me if you want to.
Dr.:	Uh huh.
Pt.:	So they said okay.
Dr.:	Are you married or you live by yourself?

Comment: A clarifying question that does not interfere with the patient's telling of his history.

Pt.:	I'm married but my wife and I are separated, see.
Dr.:	Okay, okay.
Pt.:	And, uh . . . I says, you can move in with me if you want to. So they did. Well, we moved I think the sixth day of February.
Dr.:	Yeah, this year?
Pt.:	Yeah.
Dr.:	Yeah, okay.
Pt.:	So we moved over to this little place, and, uh . . . it's about 8 weeks ago, isn't it?
Dr.:	Sure is.
Pt.:	All right, out of those 8 weeks, the God damn sister-in-law's been drunk 7 of them. And I just got to where I couldn't hardly . . .
Dr.:	And your brother-in-law? Did he drink too?
Pt.:	Oh, he drinks. He's disabled. He's drawing Social Security, welfare check, and that's what they live on.

Comment: The patient finds it more difficult to express his anger to his disabled brother-in-law than to his sister-in-law. The physician changes the subject briefly.

Dr.:	I see. What do you do for the Ajax Engineering?
Pt.:	I'm a laborer. I'm a lousy international laborers' union, North American.
Dr.:	Okay. So they are drinking a helluva lot.

Comment: As part of the rapport, the physician is using the patient's style of language. This is a way to lessen social distance. However, if you cannot comfortably use the patient's language, it may come across as being phoniness or mockery.

Pt.:	And uh . . .
Dr.:	And were you drinking at the time?
Pt.:	No.
Dr.:	How's that? You say you are an alcoholic, what do you mean you weren't drinking?

Comment: Here the physician is confronting and challenging the patient to be honest with him.

Pt.:	Well, I'm, I'm off, see? See, I'm off the booze. I just finally got where

I couldn't stand even the God damn smell of the place anymore and I went and got some whiskey.

Dr.: Okay. Now, let's stop for a minute, okay. So what I know about you is that you came from somewhere and went to work at the business down there. You moved in with your brother-in-law and sister-in-law.

Comment: The physician uses summation as a form of feedback. It tells the patient what he has heard, that he is listening, that he is interested, and how much he understands.

Pt.: Yes.

Dr.: Is this a brother-in-law from a previous marriage or something?

Pt.: Yes, my first wife. It's her brother. My first wife.

Dr.: And you moved in there because you wanted some place to stay and you didn't want to live by yourself.

Pt.: Well, like I told you Mr. . . . Doc Rusk, I'm a floater.

Dr.: You hadn't told me that yet, but I'm interested in hearing.

Pt.: Didn't I tell you I was a floater?

Dr.: Okay, so you're a floater through all your life.

Pt.: I travel all over.

Dr.: Uh huh. So you got tired of Indiana and decided you were going to go to Arizona and stopped here.

Pt.: Stopped here to visit because he [brother-in-law] used to live here and this job was a going and I thought I would just spend the winter here.

Dr.: Okay, okay, so you moved in with these people and you weren't drinking at the time you moved in.

Comment: Summation is used here to bring the patient back to the problem at hand.

Pt.: No.

Dr.: How long since you've been drinking?

Pt.: Four years.

Dr.: Now that's what I'm interested in . . .

Pt.: Now, wait a minute.

Dr.: Go ahead.

Comment: The physician allows the patient to assert himself.

Pt.: There's 1 week in that 4 years just like this.

Dr.: Yeah.

Pt.: I got on the booze once . . . it was either 2 or 3 years ago, 2 or 3 years ago, and I went to the V.A. Hospital in Illinois, went there and stayed a week.

Dr.: Uh huh.

Pt.: I came out and never touched another drop, see.

Dr.: Okay now.

Pt.: I'd seen what I was doing.

Dr.: Okay.

Pt.: I got . . .

Dr.: Now since that time 2 or 3 years ago, you haven't had a single drink of anything?

Pt.: I have had nothing.

Dr.: Not even a beer? Not even anything?

Pt.: I don't drink beer. Hell, I haven't had a beer in 6 years.

Dr.: Okay, you haven't had a drink of anything in 2 or 3 years. And then, you started drinking, when again?

Pt.: Now let's see, this is Thursday, isn't it?

Dr.: Uh huh.

Pt.: Saturday a week ago.

Dr.: Okay, about 10 days, 12 days.

Pt.: Saturday a week ago.

Dr.: Okay, do you understand why you started drinking then?

Pt.: Well, I just got so God damn disgusted with them and the smell of that beer around there all the time.

Dr.: Angry, irritated with them, angry with them!

Comment: The physician focuses on the feelings and names them.

Pt.: And I just said the hell with it. I just might just as well get drunk myself.

Dr.: They were drinking but there was other things that made you irritated at them. (Silence.) Go ahead.

Pt.: Oh, I don't know, I'm not a very smart man, Doctor Rusk. I . . .

Dr.: Don't run yourself down.

Comment: A supportive statement, said very directly with feeling, is very supportive of the patient.

Pt.: I guess you call it melancholia.

Dr.: I don't know what that is.

Comment: This is an honest statement, since the physician does not know what the patient means by "melancholia." Since patients frequently avoid communication with the use of medical terms, getting them to use other words is necessary to avoid misunderstandings.

Pt.: Isn't that the word?

Dr.: That's a nice word but I don't know what you're talking about.

Pt.: I guess you call it melancholia.

Dr.: Why don't you tell . . .

Pt.: Down in the God damn dumps.

Comment: Notice how the feelings come forth forcefully with the use of primitive terms.

Dr.: I see that, I see that, very sad.

Pt.: (Sniffs.) Just pissed off in general.

Comment: For the first time he openly acknowledges his anger.

Dr.: Okay, what were you pissed off about against them? What were they doing that was irritating as hell? There was a lot more things they were doing that you were irritated at.

Pt.: Well, I was trying to help them. I was trying to get them back on their feet. I was trying to get them to the point where a . . . they didn't have to live from just payday to payday on credit.

Dr.: Uh huh.

Pt.: See?

Dr.: Yeah.

Pt.: But all they wanted to do is drink up every damn cent.

Dr.: So you were playing a game of "I'll save you," and they didn't want to be saved.

Pt.: Well, I guess that's it.

Dr.: And they didn't want to be saved.

Pt.: (Laughs.) But I want to be. God damn it, that's why I came up here today . . .

Dr.: I don't think you're lost. I don't know, do you have to be saved? We'll get to that in a minute.

Pt.: Well, it's . . . I don't think I'm lost.

Dr.: So they got you angry. They got you angry because you wanted to save them and they said, "The hell with you, I don't want to stop drinking, I don't want to save my money either, and you just mind your own business," and it got you upset. They weren't listening to you.

Pt.: I just got pissed off and I went and got drunk, and then when I once hit that whiskey . . .

Dr.: Uh huh.

Pt.: That was it.

Dr.: Okay, now! What do you want at this point?

> **Comment:** The doctor tries to establish a mutual goal, a therapeutic contract, with the patient.

Pt.: Well . . .

Dr.: I already know, you want to stay somewhere and stop drinking and then on your way to get to Arizona.

> **Comment:** The physician could have avoided interrupting the patient by reversing the sequence of his last two statements.

Pt.: No, I'd like to get sobered up. Get this belly looked after, see what's wrong in there.

Dr.: Okay.

Pt.: There's something wrong in that belly.

Dr.: Okay.

Pt.: I don't think it's just being a drunk.

Dr.: What are you going to do after that's looked into?

Pt.: Why, I'm doing back down there and go back to work.

Dr.: Okay, now . . .

Pt.: That's how I live.

Dr.: Here's what I have to offer. That's all I have. I can't admit you to my ward. The ward we have upstairs is quite full and you're not sick enough. It's a terrible thing to say. I am glad you're not sick enough. After you have had your stomach looked into with what's hurting you, and I'll arrange to have that looked into the next half hour, okay, downstairs. If they find that you have to be hospitalized for something wrong with your stomach they'll hospitalize you. If not they won't. They will give you some advice, whatever it is, okay? Then you've got to find a place to stay. But I really don't see any reason for you to be admitted to the psychiatric ward at this point. Do you?

Comment: The physician states what help he can offer, defines a contract, and the question at the end checks with the patient as to whether or not he is in agreement.

Pt.: I don't think so either.

Dr.: Do you need anything to calm your nerves down instead of knocking off for a few days?

Pt.: Yes.

Dr.: We can arrange that.

Pt.: I need something to calm me down.

Dr.: I'll give you a prescription today. What works for you?

Pt.: I don't know.

Dr.: You've tried things before?

Pt.: They don't . . . well, I know . . .

Dr.: Nothing works as well as alcohol, but there's no end to that.

Pt.: I know I've been on . . . this one Doc gave me Librium one time and that's the only thing I know.

Dr.: Okay, fine, I'll give you that. What are you going to do with your brother-in-law, sister-in-law?

Pt.: I don't know, I don't know whether to go back there or not.

Dr.: Is that your home? You renting that? They renting that? Both of you?

Pt.: I rented the house. I paid 6 months' rent in advance. I bought the furniture.

Dr.: So why can't you kick them out if you don't like them there and you stay there?

Pt.: Why would you kick an invalid out?

Dr.: They were getting along before you got there. (A confrontation.)

Pt.: Well, they lived in a God damn rat hole.

Dr.: I don't understand.

Pt.: I tried to help them. The floors, the floors were falling out of the house.

Dr.: Wait a minute. I got a whole bunch of other people who are like that too. Are you going to take care of them too?

Pt.: No.

Dr.: I know about 500 or 600 families.

Pt.: I just couldn't see it, so I moved out.

Dr.: What are you going to do now?

Pt.: I'll go back down there and go to work.

Dr.: Yeah, but you're caught in this bind. You've got your brother-in-law, sister-in-law living in a house you've paid rent on.

Pt.: Yeah.

Dr.: You can't stand living with them.

Pt.: I can't see them living the way they do. (Laughs.)

Dr.: Yeah, what the hell you gonna do? So you drink instead, right? You forget about the whole problem by drinking. What you really want to do is kick their ass out of there and move into your own house and go to work. Isn't that what you want to do?

Comment: A restatement of the patient's expressed feeling.

Pt.: You hit it there right on the God damn head, Doc. You hit it right on the God damn head.

Dr.: What are you going to do?

Pt.: I guess I'll just go on down the road.

Dr.: Then what? Run away? (A confrontation.)

Pt.: That's all I've done for 12 years.

Dr.: When the problem gets too tough you either run away or you drink. Two ways of running away, either drinking or running away, moving, right? And you want to do the same thing again, I can't stop you. You have blown 6 months' rent.

Pt.: I may never touch another drop in 4 years.

Dr.: You may not, but how about the 6 months' rent you've put into that house down there?

Pt.: Oh nuts! What's a dollar? What's a dollar?

Dr.: Why can't you just kick them out and move in your house?

Pt.: What's a dollar?

Dr.: You're avoiding my question.

Pt.: Dollar? Dollar?

Dr.: You're avoiding my question.

Pt.: Well, you're avoiding my question, too.

> **Comment:** This exchange could easily become very hostile, but note how the physician-patient rapport can accept such a stress.

Dr.: What's a dollar?

Pt.: What's a dollar?

Dr.: One hundred cents. About 16 percent less than it was in 1964.

> **Comment:** The physician answers the question with some humor to decrease the tension and to reward the patient's assertiveness.

Pt.: Hell of a lot less than that. (Laughing as he says it.)

> **Comment:** The laugh indicates a release of anxiety developed by the previous somewhat hostile exchange.

Dr.: Now answer mine.

Pt.: It's . . . I've throwed money away all my life.

Dr.: I believe it. When do you ever do something, start acting smart and selfish and do things for yourself?

> **Comment:** A confrontation that says in part, "Be a man," and at the same time says that he is a worthwhile person who deserves more from life. Note that the physician was flexible enough not to insist immediately on an answer to his question.

Pt.: Well, I guess . . .

Dr.: Well, are you really helping them, you think? What happens when you leave and the rent ends up?

Pt.: I guess that's it. I've never done anything for myself.

> **Comment:** The patient is still reacting to the previous comment—perseveration.

Dr.: Except to run away when you chicken out.

Pt.: Say, I lived out here in 1958, I had a home.

Dr.: I don't want to talk about '58, I want to talk about right now. What happens when the 6 months is up and the rent is already gone?

Comment: Now he is directing the interview to the topic the patient wishes to avoid.

Pt.: I had a farm.

Dr.: No, look! You want to talk about that! You go find a bartender. He'll talk to you about 1958, '23 as long as you'll keep buying drinks. But it doesn't do you a bit of good—a bloody bit of good—talking about '58 or '37.

Pt.: That's when I really became, you know, a drunkard, an alcoholic.

Dr.: All we can do anything about is 1971. We can't do anything about 1958.

Pt.: Okay.

Comment: The patient is now willing to comply with the physician's request.

Dr.: What happens when your brother-in-law, sister-in-law's rent is no longer paid and the 6 months are up? What happens to them?

Pt.: Oh, they'll pay then. Oh, he'll pay it out of his check then.

Dr.: But won't it run down the same way the other house ran down?

Pt.: And uh . . . probably will.

Dr.: Okay, do you want me to let you know about that so that you can come back and save them again?

Pt.: (Laughing.) No.

Dr.: Why not? You're only good natured when you see it but you're not good natured when you don't see it. How can you be such a son-of-a-bitch as to run away and leave them like that? Shouldn't you support them for the rest of their lives?

Pt.: No.

Dr.: What's the matter with you. You dirty rat.

Pt.: (Laughs.) You rascal you. You're trying to . . .

Dr.: Put up or shut up.

Pt.: . . . make something else of it. Yeah, yeah.

Dr.: Put up or shut up. Either take care of them or don't take care of them. What is this half-ass way of running out on them? (Smiles.)

Comment: In this section of the interview the physician is aggressively confronting the patient with the idea that by helping his in-laws he is fulfilling his own needs. The physician does this by stating what the patient's behavior might be if it were exaggerated.

Pt.: You, ah . . . you're trying to turn me into an animal now, aren't you?

Dr.: No, I'm trying to turn you into a human being; you are an animal now.

Pt.: Okay.

Dr.: You've been drinking, you've been running away instead of facing the music.

Pt.: I admit that.

Dr.: I'd like to know how you are doing them any good, really. They're sitting in your house, they are drinking like hell, you're getting angrier and angrier at them, and you haven't got the guts to tell them.

Pt.: That's it, I haven't got the guts.

Dr.: And you call that acting like an animal, to walk up to them and say, "Look, you are drinking, I don't want to drink any more, I don't want to . . . you want to live in this house . . ."

Pt.: I don't have the guts to tell them.

Dr.: You want to live in this house? Fine, live in this house but you've got to stop drinking. You want to keep on drinking, then move out. Is that being an animal? It's up to you. You live your life the way you want to live it. Anything else before we quit?

Pt.: Yeah, do you think I've helped you any? (By being televised.)

Dr.: Helped me any?

Pt.: Helped you in your studies?

Dr.: I don't know. I'd like to show it (the videotape) to some other people. I don't know.

Pt.: Well, I tell you what.

Dr.: You know how I'll know. If you call me up . . . what's today, Friday?

Pt.: Yeah, no, today is Thursday.

Dr.: Thank you for helping me. Friday, Saturday, Sunday. Those are bad days for alcoholics. Weekends, because they don't work.

Pt.: Yeah.

Dr.: If you call me up Monday stone sober, say, "I'm back at work, I'm on my lunch break, I've had my talk with them, and they are moving out" or "I've had my talk with them and they have stopped drinking," then I'll know. I don't know today whether I've been of any help to you or if you've been any help to me. But Monday if you call me sometime Monday and say, "I'm not drinking any more, I'm sobered up, I'm back in my house. They said they are not going to stop drinking so until . . . Okay, you leave because . . . I'm alcoholic, and I can't have people drinking right around me." It's like putting a bottle in front of an alcoholic, which is exactly what it is. "So I can't have you in my house if you drink. I have nothing against you people drinking, if you want to drink in your house but I can't, you living the same place I'm living, where I paid the rent, if you're drinking. I'm sorry but I have to ask you to move out unless you stop." And if you've done all of that, then I'll know that you have been of help to me. I'm glad I had a chance to talk with you.

Pt.: Well, by God, I'll tell you its . . . I've had the best talk today that I've had in a long time. (Starting to cry.)

Dr.: And I think you appreciated it. It almost makes you want to cry, doesn't it?

Pt.: Yes. (Sniffing.)

Dr.: I understand. I hope it's been as helpful as you feel it is right now. You don't have to, let me say one more thing, maybe, okay! I don't think—go ahead and cry—it's okay, take your handkerchief out and cry, dammit.

Pt.: It hurts, it hurts.

Dr.: It doesn't help to bury it, it still sits inside there you know.

Pt.: It hurts though.

Dr.: Cry, take the handkerchief and cry, dammit.

Pt.: Well, I'm not ashamed to cry.

Dr.: I wish you one thing, I wish that you could like yourself more. That you didn't feel that you had to buy people to get them to like you.

Pt.: Well, I . . . I'm not buying people.

Dr.: I think you are, and I don't think you have to, you're a nice enough guy that you don't have to buy people, okay?

Pt.: Thank you.

The patient was sent home with appropriate medication after being diagnosed as having alcoholic gastritis. As was suggested in the closing of the interview, he did call back at noon on the following Monday. He was sober and had already found a job but was vague as to how the situation with his in-laws was resolved. Dr. Rusk was prevented from following this patient further because of his move from the state. In view of the fact that the physician was at times direct, assertive, confronting, and honest, it is worth noting that the patient experienced the interview with warmth and appreciation.

APPENDIXES

These appendixes have several functions. Appendix A provides the student (or anyone who is interested in improving his/her interacting skills) with exercises to work through for additional practice in the basic interactional principles presented in this text. These exercises may also be used by professional teachers as a guide for developing their own exercises to fit more precisely the needs of individual students.

Appendix B serves as a guide for learning through the videotaping of an interaction with a real or programmed (role playing) patient. The interview worksheets and interview assessment forms aid in the analysis of an interaction. The worksheet is for the interviewer to use with a recording of his/her interaction. The assessment form is for an observer to use while observing the live or recorded interaction.

Appendix C provides videotape simulations, which work very well as learning vehicles in both predoctoral and continuing education settings. They aid learning by requiring close observation of the process and content of an interaction.

From the material in these appendixes the teacher can find aids for his/her next course dealing with professional interactions in the office, the student can find additional exercises, and the health professional may have a more meaningful continuing education program at the next meeting.

APPENDIX A

COMMUNICATION EXERCISES

Statements made in the second and third person frequently are blaming or accusative; that is, the receiver of the message feels that he/she is being blames or accused of something. The receiver may then become defensive. In the professional relationship it is rare that effective (in the sense of helping the patient grow or overcome illness) communication results from putting the patient on the defensive. The following exercise is on rephrasing second- and third-person statements into first-person statements. When a speaker makes a statement in the first person ("I think. . ." or "I feel. . ."), the speaker is taking responsibility for the statement instead of being accusative.

In the following exercise read each situation and the "you" message. Then write a clear "I" message in the third column. When you have finished, compare your "I" messages with our suggestions.

Sending Messages in the First Person

Situation	*"You" message*	*"I" message*
Example: The assistant has just reported that the patient refused to restrict his diet to liquids last night. Since the restriction was crucial to the treatment of the patient, you are concerned and puzzled.	What's the matter with you, why didn't you avoid eating last night?	I feel puzzled and concerned (that I was not sensitive to your feelings) about your eating last night.
A. As a health professional, you take a chance and choose to work with a professor who is not well-liked by other students or faculty members. Surprisingly, you find your experience to be pleasing and profitable.	It turns out that you are an impressive professor, after all.	
B. An assistant corrects you regarding an error about a patient's history.	You are overstepping your bounds; would you please stop riding me?	

Continued.

Situation	"You" message	"I" message

C. A patient seems to be in a depressed mood for the entire appointment. He acts very sad. What has been the matter with you this last half hour?

> **Answers:** Any response is appropriate *if it begins with an "I" statement that communicates how "I feel."*
>
> **A.** I felt very pleased and relieved to have worked with you this summer. It makes me feel proud to see you doing so well.
>
> **B.** I feel embarrassed; I'm glad you made me aware of the error.
>
> **C.** I feel worried about your sadness right now. Is there some way I can help?
>
> *Or simply:* I feel concerned about your sadness right now.

THE LATENT CONTENT

A message usually has both a manifest and a latent content. The manifest content is the dictionary meaning of the words. The latent content is made up of the feelings—the inferred and the understood message. When interacting with another person, we may choose to react to the manifest or latent content of each message as it is sent.

In the following exercise read each patient's statement and write a *reflection* to the latent content in the column under *Receiver (professional)*. When you have finished, compare your responses with ours.

Sender (patient)	Receiver (professional)
Example: This thing has been going on for weeks. I just can't go any longer (tears) . . . I must find some way out.	You are completely exhausted, at the end of your rope, and feel you've got to find a way out.
A. Well, what about the average person who has something like what I've got. Doesn't the surgery hurt? Won't this problem come back on me anyway?	
B. I just wish someone would tell me what usually happens with the average patient who has been here with this disease.	
C. My mommy told me to come here by myself today.	

> **Answers:** **A.** You're feeling anxious and apprehensive about the discomfort you will experience, and you wonder whether the treatment is worth it.
>
> **B.** You feel irritated because we're unable to give you an answer at this time.
>
> **C.** You're feeling afraid and wish that your mother were here.

RESTATEMENT

The use of restatement (reflection or summary reply) in the receiving of a message can serve several purposes:

> 1. It can serve as an *echo* to the sender (patient) and may help the patient to continue speaking and examining his/her thoughts and actions.

2. It can enable you to *focus* the patient's attention to certain aspects of his/her *verbalizations*.
3. It can enable you to *point out* things the patient finds *difficult to verbalize*.
4. It shows that you are concerned and listening.
5. It lets the sender hear what you heard, so that it can be corrected, if necessary.
6. By your tone of voice or inflection you can emphasize some aspect of what was said, and you may thereby highlight a hidden meaning in it.

In the following exercise read each patient's statement and write a restatement in the column under *Receiver (professional)*. When you have finished, compare your responses with ours.

Sender (patient)	Receiver (professional)
Example: I'm very worried about the condition of my son.	You're very worried about him.
A. I told my wife what you said and she got kind of upset.	
B. I used to take my medicine every day, but these last few weeks I have not been able to force myself to do it regularly.	
C. I just wish somebody could tell me something for sure.	

Answers: **A.** Your wife got upset when you told her what I said.
Or Okay, she got upset.
Or simply Your wife got upset.
B. You've had difficulty in taking your medicine every day.
Or You've had difficulty in taking your medicine lately.
C. You need someone to tell you more specifically what happens to people in your situation.
Or You want to know something definite.

CLARIFICATION

Clarification is useful in understanding the patient and in letting the patient know that we really understand what he/she is saying.

In the exercise below, read each patient's statement and write a clarification in the column under *Receiver (professional)*. When you have finished, compare your responses with ours.

Sender (patient)	Receiver (professional)
Example: When I first came today, they said I will be here for a routine examination or something like that, and I really didn't know what to expect. I've been here by myself for 30 minutes. Having to wait makes me jittery.	When you first came, you thought it to be relatively simple and routine. Being here longer than you expected has lead you to become upset.
A. So then when they told me that this exercise would cure me of my problems but when I did it and it hurt, I don't	

Continued.

know about it all. I asked my friend
and he said he has never had any problems like this and he never does any
exercises. That's why I stopped.

B. Doctor, if I let you do the biopsy, I
just don't know what will happen then,
and I don't like the idea of surgery,
either. I mean, what if something happens? I feel worried about you letting
some chick give me a shot without telling me. It's all just too much to think
about. I mean, I don't know.

Answers: **A.** You thought that the discomfort from the exercise was doin
more damage than good.

B. In general, you have a lot of anxiety about the whole proce
dure.

APPENDIX B

INTERVIEW EVALUATION

Persons who are concerned with improving and maintaining their interviewing skills will be assisted by systematic feedback and evaluation. This is true for both developing students and established health professionals. Indeed, persons who are concerned with continually improving their communicative skills with their clientele may be "students" of interviewing skills throughout their professional lives.

An interview may be evaluated from several positions. The most important position is from the position of the patient. A practical method of obtaining patient evaluation is for the student to role play an interview with a programmed patient or to have an interview with a real patient. The session needs to be videotaped. Immediately after the interview the patient and the student view the videotape with a third person who acts as a facilitator.

When viewing the videotaped interview, the patient and the interviewer will probably recall many thoughts and feelings that were not said during the interview. During the interview there are many thoughts and feelings that are not voiced, because our minds work much faster than we can verbalize our feelings and thoughts. Therefore, at the beginning of the playback of the videotape, the facilitator emphasizes the ground rules that either the interviewer or patient may stop the tape any time anything comes to mind. Once the tape is stopped, the facilitator inquires as to the person's thoughts and feelings at that point. When a thought or feeling is expressed, the facilitator uses nonjudgmental, neutral, probing, understanding expressions like the following to fully understand what took place during the interview:

What were you thinking?
What did you want to say?
What were you feeling?
What had you hoped would happen?
What risks were involved in saying that?
How did you want the other person to see you?
What images did you have then? *or* What images came to mind?
What did you think the other person was feeling?
Did the other know how you were feeling?
Were you satisfied with your response? His/her response?

What got in your way of saying or doing that?

You mentioned earlier that you felt such and such; is that feeling or thought still with you (at this point on the tape)?

The second way of evaluating an interview is from the position of the interviewer. Again, the interview needs to be recorded. When videotape is available, it is preferred. In its absence audiotape is a good second choice.

To facilitate the interviewer's evaluation of an interview, we have developed the worksheet below. To use the worksheet, the interviewer assigns each of his/her replies a number in the first column. Then, using the criteria at the end of the worksheet, the interviewer analyzes the replies according to type, intent, and success. In the second column the interviewer records the letter that corresponds with the type of the reply. In the third column the interviewer records the number that corresponds with his/her intent in using the reply. What did the interviewer want to happen as a result of the reply? In the fourth column the interviewer rates the success of the reply (by listening to the patient's response to it) on a scale of 1 to 5. If the interviewer gives a low rating to a reply, he/she should place an alternate, improved reply in the fifth column.

Once the student goes over an interview in this way, he/she may then review the interview with another student or faculty person. Only through this kind of work can a person truly develop efficient interviewing skills.

INTERVIEW WORKSHEET

Reply	Type*	Intent†	Success‡	Alternate, improved reply
1				
2				
3				
4				
5				

*Type
A. Silence
B. Facilitation
C. Open-ended question
D. Support-reassurance
E. Empathy
F. Confrontation
G. Laundry-list
H. Direct question
I. Summary
J. Prescription for action
K. Statement
L. Reflection
M. Problem question
N. Interpretation
O. Bridging
P. Yes-no

†Intent
1. Focus
2. Facilitate
3. Obtain specific information
4. Change topic
5. Close off topic
6. Clarify what patient means
7. Reassure, support
8. Make a point/teach patient/state a fact
9. Stop patient's behavior
10. Obtain positive rapport
11. Tell patient what to do
12. Test patient's ability

‡Success
1. None
2. Partial
3. Acceptable
4. More than hoped for
5. Best possible choice

Reply	Type	Intent	Success	Alternate, improved reply
6				
7				
8				
9				
10				
11				
12				
13				
14				
15				
16				
17				
18				
19				
20				
21				
22				
23				
24				
25				
26				
27				
28				
29				
30				
31				
32				
33				
34				

The third way of evaluating an interview is from the position of an observer. For this type of evaluation we have developed an interview assessment form. While observing the interview or the recording of the interview, the observer fills out the form, which is then used for discussion and review with the interviewer. It may also be filed as a record of the progress of the student during a course of study.

The form covers the nonverbal as well as the verbal aspects of the interaction. It focuses on the interview process as well as the content of information obtained by the process.

_____   _____
       Date   Name of interviewer

INTERVIEW ASSESSMENT FORM

	Needs improvement	Acceptable	Well done
Approaches patient			
Greeting, use of name	☐	☐	☐
Seating, physical setting	☐	☐	☐
Degree of control	☐	☐	☐
Purpose of interview	☐	☐	☐

COMMENT:

Begins biography of problem*			
Facilitates beginning comments	☐	☐	☐
Open-ended questions	☐	☐	☐
Silence	☐	☐	☐

COMMENT:

Continues chronicle*			
Support	☐	☐	☐
Reassurance	☐	☐	☐
Empathy	☐	☐	☐
Confrontation	☐	☐	☐
Reflection	☐	☐	☐
Silence	☐	☐	☐
Summary	☐	☐	☐
Nonverbal	☐	☐	☐

COMMENT:

_____
*Each item within the section may or may not be used during an interview.

	Needs improvement	*Acceptable*	*Well done*

Directs for diagnostic details*

	Needs improvement	Acceptable	Well done
Direct questions	☐	☐	☐
Laundry lists	☐	☐	☐
Yes-no questions	☐	☐	☐
Suggestive questions	☐	☐	☐
Why questions	☐	☐	☐

COMMENT:

Elucidates each problem

	Needs improvement	Acceptable	Well done
Location	☐	☐	☐
Quality	☐	☐	☐
Quantity	☐	☐	☐
Chronology	☐	☐	☐
Physical-biologic	☐	☐	☐
Psychosocial	☐	☐	☐
Aggravating and alleviating factors	☐	☐	☐

COMMENT:

Finalizes and closes

	Needs improvement	Acceptable	Well done
Summary	☐	☐	☐
Closure	☐	☐	☐

COMMENT:

Quality of relationship

	Needs improvement	Acceptable	Well done
Control	☐	☐	☐
Associates to patient's words	☐	☐	☐
Feelings toward patient	☐	☐	☐
Acceptance	☐	☐	☐
Concern	☐	☐	☐
Interest	☐	☐	☐
Feelings from patient	☐	☐	☐

COMMENT:

---

*Each item within the section may or may not be used during an interview.

Continued.

Report by interviewer (after interview)

	Needs improvement	Acceptable	Well done
Verbal observations	☐	☐	☐
Nonverbal observations	☐	☐	☐

COMMENT:

Summary of interview (critique)

_____

Signature of observer

APPENDIX C

VIDEOTAPE SIMULATIONS

The videotape simulation is a most useful technique for helping a student learn about the personal communication interactions in professional situations and how to develop in the professional role to which he/she is striving.

This technique combines role playing, videotape, self-confrontation, group support, and group learning. An article by Froelich and Bishop, "One Plus One Equals Three,"* describes this technique. The title emphasizes that the outcome in learning is more than what one would expect from just combining role playing and videotape.

A simulation that has been used with students is provided in this appendix as an illustration. Members of the class or group are selected to play each role. If persons who are not involved in the class or group are used, the discussion involvement in the simulation is markedly reduced.

The simulation is titled, "Difficult Patient". The first part of the instructions names the role players and gives the setting of the problem. This information is given to each role player.

The role players meet to make the videotape outside of the class period or meeting. They each review the statement of the situation. Then each role player is given his/her special instructions concerning the role he/she is playing. The role players are instructed not to share any information about what is in their special instructions.

After the role players have had 5 minutes to read their instructions, the role play begins. The first scene is of the patient and receptionist. The other role players are not allowed to see or hear what happens during this interaction. The interaction is taped for from 2 to 6 minutes—as long as it is productive. The simulation then goes on to the next logical interaction, probably a conversation between the patient and the physician associate. During this interaction, the persons playing the nurse and the physician are not allowed to hear what is going on.

Next scene will be between the patient, physician, nurse, and physician associate. The final scene is between the physician and the staff either in the office or another room, depending on how it would most naturally occur.

---

*Froelich, R. E. and Bishop, F. M.: One Plus One Equals Three, Medical and Biological Illustration, 19(1):15-18, 1969.

The total time on the videotape is usually about 20 to 30 minutes. A simulation of this length provides plenty of material for a 2- to 4-hour class discussion.

It is best to have an interval of at least 24 hours between the taping and the discussion. Such a time interval allows the role players to become less defensive about the role they played and leads to more open discussion and learning. At the beginning of class each student is given a copy of the statement of the situation, and the class discusses the problems that are inherent in the situation for at least 5 minutes before the tape is started. Once the tape has been started, anyone can stop the tape at any time by saying "stop." The discussion about what has been seen then begins. The learning comes from the discussion, *not* from the tape. In fact, after class, the tape should be erased because it is of little value once the class has gone over it. It will not work with next year's class. They need to make their own tape.

Thus, the session consists of viewing 20 seconds to 2 minutes of tape, discussing it for 10 to 15 minutes, viewing more tape, and so on. It is a fun way to teach, and the discussion is at the particular level of the group's interest and understanding. It works with nonprofessionals and advanced specialists; the only difference is in the level of the discussion that develops.

Following this illustration are the first pages of several other simulations. Make up your own individual specific instructions for these. If you are unable to come up with specific instructions you may write R. E. Froelich and F. M. Bishop for copies.

DIFFICULT PATIENT

Mr. Colwill has come to his family physician's office and is telling the receptionist that he had an appointment to see the doctor. In fact, he does not have an appointment, but is quite convincing and demanding.

Mr. Colwill has a past medical history of diabetes with frequent complaints of infection, poor sugar control, and peripheral neuropathy. He has also had polio with some residual weakness in his lower extremeties, and he lost three fingers on his left hand in a home workshop accident. Recently, instead of consulting his family physician, he has seen a urologist and an internist specializing in infectious diseases; his wife has seen a gynecologist for abdominal pain. Mr. Colwill has had broken appointments for routine follow-up and the physician's staff has been irritated by his demands and unkept appearance.

In the last few years as part of his rehabilitation he has been trained and worked as an administrative assistant in the local school of medicine. From this position he personally knows many physicians.

The receptionist is Ms. Richards who has worked for Dr. Michael for 4 years. Dr. Michael is the family physician. Howard Adams is the physician associate working with Dr. Michael. Ms. Norman is the office nurse.

Mr. Colwill has an abscess in his right axilla, which is painful and interfering with his working.

Ms. Richards, receptionist

Mr. Colwill is really forcing you to get his records and demanding to see Dr. Michael. You try to have him see one of the residents or the physician's assistant, but he will have none of it. You know that Dr. Michael has to give a talk at noon and plans to review it now, but you have to inform him that Mr. Colwill demands to see him. You feel that somehow you should not have had to do this, but you could not alter Mr. Colwill's demands.

Elaborate in any way you choose. Use your training, your experience, your imagination, your perception of the situation. Remember, our aim is to uncover as many as possible of the issues involved in the physician's and the staff's responsibility to the patient.

Howard Adams, physician associate

You have had experience with Mr. Colwill before. He does not respect you and always wants to pull rank on you by demanding to see the doctor. You know that you can evaluate an abscess in the axilla, its extent, depth, and whether or not any nerves are involved in the inflammation. You feel that you should see Mr. Colwill and that Dr. Michael should not be bothered until after you have done a physical examination of the area and extremity involved.

Elaborate in any way you choose. Use your training, your experience, your imagination, your perception of the situation. Remember, our aim is to uncover as many as possible of the issues involved in the physician's and the staff's responsibility to the patient.

Ms. Norman, office nurse

You have been with Dr. Michael for 15 years. You have known Mr. Colwill almost that long. He has been a problem all of that time. You feel that he acts like an angry child and have strong feelings how you would like to see him managed. So far he has not been managed in the way you would like. At this point you would prefer not to have to bother with him. But being a dedicated person you do your job as you must.

Elaborate in any way you choose. Use your training, your experience, your imagination, your perception of the situation. Remember, our aim is to uncover as many as possible of the issues involved in the physician's and the staff's responsibility to the patient.

Dr. Michael

Mr. Colwill irritates your staff and you. He has not shaven in two days, he has broken appointments you have made for him, he goes to other physicians without even letting you know about it. You hear about whom he has seen at hospital staff meetings. None of the doctors want to treat him because of his failure to follow orders.

This noon you have an important talk to present for your medical center staff, you planned to review the talk right now—just at the time Mr. Colwill demands to see you.

Elaborate in any way you choose. Use your training, your experience, your imagination, your perception of the situation. Remember, our aim is to uncover as many as possible of the issues involved in the physician's responsibility to the patient.

POSTPARTUM PATIENT

Mrs. Owens, a 25-year-old female, with a 3-year-old daughter, delivered a term male yesterday at 2:00 P.M. This morning, she refused to feed the baby boy. Ms. Bloom, the nursing student assigned to Mrs. Owens this morning, just reviewed the chart and is about to see the patient.

Mrs. King, the nursing instructor has 6 nursing students on the ward, which is quite active. They had 5 deliveries yesterday and have 2 patients in labor now. Mrs. Field, a social worker, is assigned to work with the OB patients and is on the unit to see another patient.

DIAGNOSTIC PROBLEM

Mr. Williams, a 50-year-old hardware store owner and operator, has had a cough for some time. Two or 3 months ago he noticed a lump at the right base of his neck while shaving. It is still present. He is seeing Dr. King, his family physician, for evaluation of the lump. Dr. King has the ability and facilities to biopsy and diagnose the tissue from the lesion.

Mrs. Williams is 46 years old, helps in the hardware store part-time, keeps the books, and is the mother of John (20) and Bob (18). The family is planning an extended trip through Europe next summer. Because of the business Mr. Williams has not had a vacation for 6 years, but recently hired an assistant who should be able to take over the business by summer. Mr. Williams' life-long ambition has been to travel and especially visit with his family the places he saw in Europe during World War II.

Dr. Sewell is a thoracic surgeon who has consulted with Dr. King on a number of patient problems.

SERIOUS ILLNESS

Dr. Arnold is the youngest physician in his community. Mrs. Long is an attractive, 21-year-old who has never been sick or hospitalized. She comes to Dr. Arnold because of no menstrual periods for 2 months and because of increasing fatigue over the last 2 weeks. She has been unable to climb a flight of steps without stopping for breath. She noted that she bruised very easily 3 days ago when she bumped into a chair. Mr. Long, an electrician, brought her to the office. They have been married 10 months. After the physical examination, which showed marked pallor and confirmed the diagnosis of a 3-month pregnancy, Mrs. Long was admitted to the hospital for laboratory studies. Mrs. Long reacted to the pain of each drawing of blood, which concerned the technician. Initial studies showed a 5 gram hemoglobin.

Dr. Arnold has had a consultation with the hematologist, Dr. Harold, who has confirmed the initial diagnosis. Dr. Arnold has not yet discussed the diagnosis with Mrs. Long or with her husband.

IRREGULAR PERIODS

Patricia Parker is a 16-year-old daughter of Dr. William Parker, a family physician. Mrs. Parker took Patricia to see Dr. Obert, a gynecologist, because of irregular menstrual periods. Dr. Obert did a physical examination including a Pap smear. The Pap smear was questionable so on a repeat visit a biopsy was obtained. The results of the biopsy and other examinations have just been reviewed by Dr. Obert. He must now transmit the information to those concerned. The remainder of the physical examination was within normal limits.

In addition to Patricia, there are three younger siblings, two girls and a boy. Patricia enjoys the family and looks forward to a future in art which she can combine with raising a family. Patricia has a steady boy friend.

ALCOHOLIC

Mr. George Mayer is a 38-year-old city councilman who is up for election in 6 weeks as mayor of the city of 50,000 in a farming area. Dr. Russell has heard a colleague discuss the management of Mr. Mayer as an alcoholic, but has not treated him before. There has also been a rumor that Mr. Mayer directed city funds to a housing project in which he was part owner.

Mr. Mayer's doctor is out of town for a week. This Sunday morning Dr. Russell is on call and is called to the emergency room to see Mr. Mayer who is sick at his stomach, has unsteady gait, a gross tremor of his hands, and a headache. His eyes are bloodshot, his skin shows signs of dehydration; he hasn't shaven in 2 days, and he has the odor of alcohol on his breath. Dr. Russell is concerned that Mr. Mayer is showing signs of pending D.T.'s.

Dr. Russell recommends to Mr. Mayer's brother and father that the patient be hospitalized, but their first reaction was to refuse hospitalization for fear that the news would get to the press and ruin his future public life. Hospitalization would also prevent him from getting to his speaking engagement Tuesday evening. To complicate Dr. Russell's position, Mr. Mayer is of the opposite political party. Dr. Russell has contributed to the campaign fund of Mr. Mayer's opponent.

WARD MANAGEMENT PROBLEM

Mrs. Jones, a 34-year-old married female was admitted to the psychiatric ward two weeks ago because of an episode during which she threatened her husband with a gun. She has been very negativistic, but has slowly become more cooperative until today. Since admission, resident "A" has seen her daily. He is out of the hospital when the patient suddenly demands to be given papers to sign herself out of the hospital.

It is not clear why she wants to sign out. The ward nurse believes it is just part of her character pattern. The patient was noted by a technician to have had an argument with another patient this morning. Resident "B," a second year resident, is on call and comes to the ward. Before he arrives, the social worker who has seen the patient's husband arrives on the ward. She saw the husband yesterday and learned that he is having trouble caring for the children and has been seeing a great deal of a divorced neighbor lady since the patient has been hospitalized.

Resident "A" believes that the patient is depressed, suicidal, and has very severe inferiority feelings associated with suspiciousness. The resident dates the onset of the patient's difficulty back to her association with her hostile, demanding father.

The ward physician expressed the belief shortly after admission that the patient has an acting-out character disorder.

MASTECTOMY

Mrs. Johnson is now in her third day after a radical mastectomy for a cancer in her right breast. Today is the first day back in her room, the first day she has felt like talking. Prior to surgery, she did not know whether or not she had cancer. She was told that a cancer was found and that a radical mastectomy was performed. Because of the large bandage, she has no idea of her appearance; all she knows is that she is very sore and that it is painful to move.

Mrs. Johnson has 3 children aged 12, 8, and 5 years. Her husband runs a small retail business which is open long hours.

INDEX

J

Jargon, 39
Judgment, 49

L

Laundry-list question, 24, 95, 100, 107
Laver, J., 54

M

"Make meaning," 3, 4
Marital history, 106
Mathematical ability, 48
Memory, 49
Mental status, 47
"Message in receiver," 5, 21, 37
Multiple questions, 38

O

Office setting, 86
Open-ended question, 11, 92, 93, 94, 98, 99,
   100, 107
Opening statement, 9, 75
Orientation, 49

P

Parting, physical, 41
Panic, 14, 172
Patient
   crying, 20, 109, 140, 141, 173, 177, 180
   defensive, 120
   fearful, 112
   gifts from, 139
   manipulation, 136
   question, 34, 121, 128, 129
   testing, 128, 141
   trust, 70, 73
Posture, body, 53, 58
Preinterview data, 6, 7
Prescription for action, 41
Probing question, 26
Problem question, 48, 49

Q

Question
   antagonizing, 29, 32, 101
   direct, 25, 99, 105, 107
   laundry-list, 24, 95, 100, 107
   multiple, 38
   open-ended, 11, 92, 93, 94, 98, 99, 100, 107
   patient, 34, 121, 128, 129
   probing, 26
   problem, 48, 49

suggestive, 33, 38
"why," 32
"yes-no," 32, 38, 123

R

Reassurance, 13, 39, 100
Receptionist, 82
Referral
   of patient, 42
   to psychiatrist, 43
Reflection, 17, 92, 93, 94, 103, 108, 112, 173
Ritchey, H. M., 144
Rusk, T. N., 172

S

Sensorium, 48-50
Shaking hands, 85
Silence, 19, 38
Sorrow, 65-67, 81
Sources of data, 8
Statement
   accusative, 76, 77
   blaming, 77
   bridging, 28, 96, 98, 105
   compliant, 76
   final, 41
   healthy, 77
   intellectual, 77
   irrelevant, 77
   opening, 9, 75
Stroke, management of, 75
Suggestive question, 33, 38
Suicide, 51, 103, 104, 144, 146
Summation, 22, 94, 98, 99, 141, 176
Support, 13, 15, 100, 110, 177

T

Therapeutic contract, 10, 144, 149, 177
Topic
   change of, 27
   closing, 15
Touch, 21, 128

V

Verwoerdt, A., 13, 38
Voice, 53

W

Wexler, M., 13, 16, 18, 25
"Why" question, 32

Y

"Yes-no" question and answer, 32, 38, 123